A dissertation on the motion of the blood, and on the effects of bleeding. Verified by experiments made on living animals. To which are added, observations on the heart, ... By ... Dr. Alb. Haller, ... Translated by a physician.

Albrecht von Haller

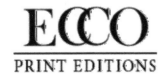

A dissertation on the motion of the blood, and on the effects of bleeding. Verified by experiments made on living animals. To which are added, observations on the heart, ... By ... Dr. Alb. Haller, ... Translated by a physician.
Haller, Albrecht von
ESTCID: N000002
Reproduction from Harvard University Houghton Library

London : printed for J. Whiston and B. White, 1757.
iv,156p. ; 8°

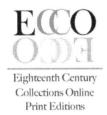

Eighteenth Century
Collections Online
Print Editions

Gale ECCO Print Editions

Relive history with *Eighteenth Century Collections Online*, now available in print for the independent historian and collector. This series includes the most significant English-language and foreign-language works printed in Great Britain during the eighteenth century, and is organized in seven different subject areas including literature and language; medicine, science, and technology; and religion and philosophy. The collection also includes thousands of important works from the Americas.

The eighteenth century has been called "The Age of Enlightenment." It was a period of rapid advance in print culture and publishing, in world exploration, and in the rapid growth of science and technology – all of which had a profound impact on the political and cultural landscape. At the end of the century the American Revolution, French Revolution and Industrial Revolution, perhaps three of the most significant events in modern history, set in motion developments that eventually dominated world political, economic, and social life.

In a groundbreaking effort, Gale initiated a revolution of its own: digitization of epic proportions to preserve these invaluable works in the largest online archive of its kind. Contributions from major world libraries constitute over 175,000 original printed works. Scanned images of the actual pages, rather than transcriptions, recreate the works ***as they first appeared.***

Now for the first time, these high-quality digital scans of original works are available via print-on-demand, making them readily accessible to libraries, students, independent scholars, and readers of all ages.

For our initial release we have created seven robust collections to form one the world's most comprehensive catalogs of 18th century works.

Initial Gale ECCO Print Editions collections include:

> ***History and Geography***
> Rich in titles on English life and social history, this collection spans the world as it was known to eighteenth-century historians and explorers. Titles include a wealth of travel accounts and diaries, histories of nations from throughout the world, and maps and charts of a world that was still being discovered. Students of the War of American Independence will find fascinating accounts from the British side of conflict.

Social Science
Delve into what it was like to live during the eighteenth century by reading the first-hand accounts of everyday people, including city dwellers and farmers, businessmen and bankers, artisans and merchants, artists and their patrons, politicians and their constituents. Original texts make the American, French, and Industrial revolutions vividly contemporary.

Medicine, Science and Technology
Medical theory and practice of the 1700s developed rapidly, as is evidenced by the extensive collection, which includes descriptions of diseases, their conditions, and treatments. Books on science and technology, agriculture, military technology, natural philosophy, even cookbooks, are all contained here.

Literature and Language
Western literary study flows out of eighteenth-century works by Alexander Pope, Daniel Defoe, Henry Fielding, Frances Burney, Denis Diderot, Johann Gottfried Herder, Johann Wolfgang von Goethe, and others. Experience the birth of the modern novel, or compare the development of language using dictionaries and grammar discourses.

Religion and Philosophy
The Age of Enlightenment profoundly enriched religious and philosophical understanding and continues to influence present-day thinking. Works collected here include masterpieces by David Hume, Immanuel Kant, and Jean-Jacques Rousseau, as well as religious sermons and moral debates on the issues of the day, such as the slave trade. The Age of Reason saw conflict between Protestantism and Catholicism transformed into one between faith and logic -- a debate that continues in the twenty-first century.

Law and Reference
This collection reveals the history of English common law and Empire law in a vastly changing world of British expansion. Dominating the legal field is the *Commentaries of the Law of England* by Sir William Blackstone, which first appeared in 1765. Reference works such as almanacs and catalogues continue to educate us by revealing the day-to-day workings of society.

Fine Arts
The eighteenth-century fascination with Greek and Roman antiquity followed the systematic excavation of the ruins at Pompeii and Herculaneum in southern Italy; and after 1750 a neoclassical style dominated all artistic fields. The titles here trace developments in mostly English-language works on painting, sculpture, architecture, music, theater, and other disciplines. Instructional works on musical instruments, catalogs of art objects, comic operas, and more are also included.

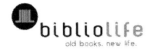

The BiblioLife Network

This project was made possible in part by the BiblioLife Network (BLN), a project aimed at addressing some of the huge challenges facing book preservationists around the world. The BLN includes libraries, library networks, archives, subject matter experts, online communities and library service providers. We believe every book ever published should be available as a high-quality print reproduction; printed on-demand anywhere in the world. This insures the ongoing accessibility of the content and helps generate sustainable revenue for the libraries and organizations that work to preserve these important materials.

The following book is in the "public domain" and represents an authentic reproduction of the text as printed by the original publisher. While we have attempted to accurately maintain the integrity of the original work, there are sometimes problems with the original work or the micro-film from which the books were digitized. This can result in minor errors in reproduction. Possible imperfections include missing and blurred pages, poor pictures, markings and other reproduction issues beyond our control. Because this work is culturally important, we have made it available as part of our commitment to protecting, preserving, and promoting the world's literature.

GUIDE TO FOLD-OUTS MAPS and OVERSIZED IMAGES

The book you are reading was digitized from microfilm captured over the past thirty to forty years. Years after the creation of the original microfilm, the book was converted to digital files and made available in an online database.

In an online database, page images do not need to conform to the size restrictions found in a printed book. When converting these images back into a printed bound book, the page sizes are standardized in ways that maintain the detail of the original. For large images, such as fold-out maps, the original page image is split into two or more pages

Guidelines used to determine how to split the page image follows:

• Some images are split vertically; large images require vertical and horizontal splits.
• For horizontal splits, the content is split left to right.
• For vertical splits, the content is split from top to bottom.
• For both vertical and horizontal splits, the image is processed from top left to bottom right.

A DISSERTATION

ON THE

MOTION of the BLOOD,

AND ON THE

EFFECTS of BLEEDING.

VERIFIED BY

EXPERIMENTS made on Living Animals.

To which are added,

OBSERVATIONS on the HEART, proving that IRRITABILITY is the primary Cause of its Motion.

By the Celebrated

DR. ALB. HALLER,

President of the Royal Society of Sciences at GOTTINGEN, Member of the Royal Academy of Sciences at PARIS, Fellow of the Royal Societies of LONDON, BERLIN, STOCKHOLM, &c

Translated by a PHYSICIAN.

LONDON:

Printed for J. WHISTON and B. WHITE, in Fleet-street.

MDCCLVII.

THE

PREFACE.

THE learned author of this dissertation presented it to the Royal Society at GOTTINGEN, the eighth day of October, 1754; and it is published in the fourth volume of the Transactions of that learned assembly. He calls it an Analytical Exposition of Results; and these he hath verified by two hundred and thirty-five experiments made on living animals. Hereunto is added a short

short dissertation, containing the author's experiments made on the heart, proving that irritability is the primary cause of its motion. A translation of the experiments themselves, as presented to the said society, the twenty-sixth of March, 1756, and which are the foundation of this dissertation, will be very soon published.

ON THE

CIRCULATION of the BLOOD.

YOU will excuse, good firs, my laſt year's ſilence, if you conſider my ſudden and unexpected departure, the length of the voyage, the difficulty of conveying my books, the fatigue of a new eſtabliſhment, and laſtly an unhappy fall that deprived me for many months of the uſe of an arm, I did not, notwithſtanding all this, forget you nor the duties I owe you: and indeed how could I forget you, with whom I have paſſed my time ſo agreeably? you who, by your ſtrict union and continued labours during the laſt years of my reſidence at Gottingen, gave me much pleaſure and ſatisfaction? and laſtly you, gentlemen, whoſe friendſhip is a ſenſible part of my happineſs, the abſence whereof, I have always regarded as an irreparable loſs? Could I forget my duty when called upon, and by an honourable office our prudent protector had been pleased to preserve for me, and through my desire of enquiring after truth? could I forget a society, to whose business I ought justly to submit, since I enjoy its honours? For these reasons, gentlemen, I have been considering what subject I could make choice of, that would equally come under your cognizance as well as mine, having changed my course of study as to the anatomy of the human body. I think now the only thing remaining for me, is the dissecting of living animals. I have opened a great number at Gottingen, an account whereof I have in my papers, and have added thereto dissections that I made at Berne, to divert me, by the study of sciences, from other business of civil life that is less engaging. To these dissections, I add microscopical observations of cold animals, one hundred whereof I have sacrificed to my enquiries, partly with Dr. Remus and others, since my return into the country. I shall take another opportunity of informing you what experiments have taught me concerning respiration and generation, and here I shall only take notice of the nature of the arteries and veins, the globules of blood, their motion in the vessels, the causes of this motion, the changes that ligatures and bleeding can produce therein, and occasionally

sionally the changes the blood can undergo. These several articles I propose as the subject-matter of as many chapters.

CHAP. I.

Concerning the Structure of the Arteries and Veins.

I Have not very attentively examined the great vessels of animals that have cold blood, yet having observed the Aorta to go out double from a thick solid trunk and cellular internally, I traced it even to the Mesentery, and I observed the pulmonary arteries, which are not large, and are only of a diameter proportional to that of this viscus, to arise from the descending branch. I apprehended this viscus somewhat like a bladder for swimming, each lobe inclosing a considerable cavity, whose circumference is surrounded by a series of polygon vesicles, interspersed with little arteries, agreeable to Malpighy's description of the same, they differ from the vesicles of the lungs of men, by their magnitude and by their angular figure, and are themselves surrounded by other vesicles much smaller, which one can hardly distinguish, and which are not always seen, and which render the lungs of frogs somewhat like those of man.

In the Mesentery of these animals, the arterial trunks extend themselves direct enough towards the Intestines, where they divide and spread themselves in a serpentine manner upon their surface, or uniting themselves one with another, they make rings resembling those which the colic and ileocolic artery form on the human Colon. We can see distinctly, in these ramifications, that the total of the lights and cavities of two branches from one trunk, is greater than the light of the trunk itself, and as far as I could observe with a microscope, the arteries in the Mesentery are conical: although during the time the animal suffers under the experiment, their diameter may be often changed and disfigured, and undergo different strangulations, as the blood is propelled more towards one place than another.

The veins almost like the arteries, exceed them in number and diameter, which is almost double that of the arteries, but the chief difference of these two kinds of vessels, is in the network of the veins Their trunks subdivide themselves successively into very small ramifications of the diameter of a single globule, and mixing themselves with other veins of the Mesentery, form a venal network, without any one
branch

branch of an artery (a) These veins are apparently cylindrical, with frequent flexions, their angles of re-union are pretty large, and the areas that separate them are polygons, somewhat resembling a square. Generally speaking, I have not observed in my experiments, any arteries of a globule diameter, because perhaps the thickness of the membranes hinders one from perceiving the faint redness of a single globule, the apparent white colour of these small vessels confounds them, with the membranes on which they creep, the great arteries themselves are pale when the veins appear very red, without any mixture of blue As to the tails of fish, I have sometimes observed between two parallel arteries, arterial plexuses, whose vessels appeared of the size of a globule of blood.

On examining carefully the membranes of the arteries, they will be found thick, white, and compact. Their thickness hath not always the same appearance with the whole diameter of the artery, and this thickness often makes one half of the diameter, and the cavity of the canal the other half: sometimes it makes the greater part of it. It happens that the blood is propelled with more force in the arteries, without any

---

(a) D. Heide de Sang Missione, p 8 & Lewenhoeck Cont. Arcan. Nat 3. p 62 speak of this network.

dilation of the whole diameter, becaufe the blood poffeffeth the greater part of their light, and the parieties of the arteries are reduced to a third or a fourth part of their firft thicknefs. By this it appears, that the denfity of the arteries increafeth in proportion to the force with which the blood is propelled therein. The greater fpace the blood poffeffeth in a circle, the lefs remains for the parieties, and confequently the more the fibres of thefe parieties muft be compreffed. This, if I miftake not, helps us to account for the hardnefs of the pulfe in fome fevers, yet not that I would exclude the blood's increafed denfity

All like the arterial tube may be full beyond meafure, but it may happen alfo that a fufficient fulnefs may be wanting. Nothing happens more frequent than to find in frogs empty veins, and alfo arteries either quite or half empty, or even which contain not more than one, two, or three columns of blood globules, and it is not confonant to experiments, to believe that the veffels contracted in proportion to the quantity of blood they contain are always full, and that they only become narrower when they contain but little blood: for although fafting diminifhes the quantity of blood, yet the diameter of the blood-veffels is not leffened, and often bleeding or other caufes, re-eftablifhes the

the course of the blood that was suspended in some arteries, thereby restoring to them their former plenitude.

But there is another change in the diameter of the artery that frequently happens, and which I have often produced by pricking the artery, and which at other times, I have observed to happen from some cause unknown to me; I mean the true Aneurisme which is found so often in the arteries of frogs examined with a microscope, and which is a tumour almost oval, which the superior part of an artery supplies with blood, which blood this tumor conveys to the inferior part of the same trunk. I disagree with some authors who are of opinion, that the true Aneurisme ought to be excluded from the number of chirurgical maladies *(b)*. I have seen it happen, as I have before related, from some cause unknown to me *(c)*; and I have since learned how to produce it at pleasure For this purpose, I separate the two laminæ of the Mesentery from the two coats of an artery, after which I shake it, so as entirely to disengage it from its connecting cellular substance; after this I soon find an Aneurisme produced. It is

(b) See on this dispute Dr Friend's History of Physic, p 184. the quarto edition of Paris 1735

(c) These Aneurisms Lewenhoeck saw, when he declared the vessels grew thicker, where the blood began to coagulate.

also equally formed after an incision, and especially after the pricking of the artery. Sometimes also, though not so often, the like tumours are observed in the veins; but chiefly in these we find, as I have a little before related, inequalities in their diameters, which is the reason that that part which is nearest the heart, is not always the largest.

I have not perceived small vessels upon the membranes of the arteries, but in frogs there is often found on the membranes that compose the vessels of every order, particular black spots a little like arrows, formed in network, the cause whereof seems very uncertain. The veins have so delicately thin a membrane, that one may see very distinctly the blood globules; they seem to form a kind of chain like a row of beads, somewhat like Cowper *(d)* and Cheselden's *(e)* descriptions of the small vessels, but the course of these vessels they take no notice of. This made Lewenhoeck say, that the blood-vessels have no membranes, and that the red globules make their own way into the places where they find the least resistance *(f)*. I have never yet observed any valve in the veins of frogs.

I have never been able, even by the help of a microscope, to discover any muscular

(d) Append. ad Bidl. t. 3. fol. 3.
(e) Anatomy of Human Body, edit. 6. t. 3.
(f) Experiments and Contemp. p. 184.

fibre

fibre in the veſſels of the Meſentery, altho' the veins near the heart are certainly provided with them; for we can very diſtinctly obſerve in both Venæ cavæ motions of conſtriction correſponding to thoſe of the auricle

Thoſe red ſpots occaſioned by extravaſated blood, taken notice of upon all kind of veſſels after wounds, and eſpecially upon the human arteries after an inflammation; theſe ſpots, I ſay, demonſtratively prove that all theſe veſſels are accompanied with ſome cellular ſubſtance, which, by reaſon of its tranſparency when empty, eſcapes our view. It is not uncommon to ſee capillary veins, lying connected upon the arteries in the major part of their courſe, and without interrupting in the leaſt the motion of their fluids, and this teacheth us how little we ought to regard the reaſon that is given, why the left ſpermatic vein is inſerted into the Emulgent rather than into the Cava. It is, ſay they, a precaution of nature, leaſt the pulſations of the Aorta ſhould obſtruct the cavity of ſo ſmall a vein, or diſorder the courſe of its blood. The weakneſs of this theory may be again proved by the human Aorta, which, in all the cavity of the breaſt, is ſurrounded with ſmall veins ariſing from the ſuperior Intercoſtal, and yet notwithſtanding their being ſo near ſo large a veſſel, receive

thereby

thereby no detriment to their functions. Hereupon may be consulted the description and figures, that I have published of the bronchial artery.

I have not traced in frogs the small vessels which form the continuations between the arteries and the veins. The Mesenteries of these animals are not proper for this observation, because this union seems to be made in the membranes of the Intestines, which are too opaque for observation: but this is very distinctly seen in fish, and as I have in a manner observed nothing but what is already known, I shall be short on this article. In the tail of some small fish we see four little bones, each whereof is accompanied with an artery and a vein. The conveyance of blood from the one to the other, is made in two different manners, often the artery bends itself even to the extremity of the tail, and bending like a hook, turns parallel to itself. By this simple method, a number of arteries, even of the diameter of many globules (*g*), become veins: therefore it is no wonder if air, sewet, and in general the liquors injected by anatomists, find so easy a passage through the lungs, reins, Mesentery, heart, and even the human brain, and pass from the arteries

(*g*) Lewenhoeck's Experim. and Contem. t. 11 p. 177, limits the number to three, but I have seen the contrary.

of these viscera into their corresponding veins. This is the first method of union, described by Lewenhoeck in different parts of his works (*h*). There is yet another method more complex, it proceeds from an artery under different angles; many branches of one, two, or three globules diameter terminating themselves in a parallel vein, supply it with arterial blood. This last manner of communication, is as often observed in fish as the first. This Lewenhoeck hath spoken of (*i*).

What remains for me now to enquire after, is what the vessels are which Dr. Boerhaave (*k*) appoints for the conveying of the liquids thinner than blood. A person not accustomed to observation, easily persuades himself he sees them, when he observes for that purpose, in the Mesentery of frogs, little vessels which suffer only a yellow globule to pass them. Deceived by this colour, I thought myself happy some years ago, in having it in my power to make this observation, and Mr. Baker (*l*) mentions the same error in a friend of his but an observer less subject to believe what he desires, does not long enjoy this pleasure, and soon

(*h*) Ibid p. 106. f 6 A f 10
(*i*) Γ Sive Exper & Contem p 178 f 1 p 183 f. 14 p 185 f 15 p 186 f 16 17. and in other places.
(*k*) De Usu ratiocinii mecanici, p 14.
(*l*) Microscope made easy, p 136.

confesseth that all he saw, were only very small veins arising from red veins, which uniting become again red veins, containing only red globules. If to the eye they appear yellow, it is only because the colour of a single row of globules being extremely weak, vanishes and dischargeth itself through the membranes, and is not apparent to us, until the globules become more numerous. The eminent M Senac and an anonymous author, have mentioned this before (n).

Notwithstanding this, I will not advance that there are no vessels smaller than the red ones, all that I establish is, that I have observed nothing that contradicts a possibility of their being arteries, and canals, containing a liquor different from blood, and that there may be other vessels appointed for the circulation of a thinner fluid, for we observe them, in the muscles of eels of a silver colour, containing a humour different from the blood. There are many other reasons to confirm this opinion

(n) Lettre sur le Nouveau Système de la Voix p 55

CHAP.

CHAP. II.

Of the Humours.

IT remains for me now to speak of the fluids contained in the arteries and veins. Of these I have hitherto observed two kinds, the red globules and an invisible liquid in frogs and fish, which is called in large animals by the name of lymph or serosity. I will begin with the red globules, the discovery whereof seems to me to be owing to Malpighy, although he (*a*) considered them in a different light. What I call globules are little lentils red or yellow; frogs and fish have them of both these colours. They are yellow in animals becoming feeble, and are of a deeper red on the animal's recovering strength; and this redness doth not solely depend, as some authors imagine (*b*),

(*a*) In his treatise De Omento & Adiposis Ductibus, which he published in 1665, he describes, p. 42 of the London edition, a blood vessel of the Omentum, in which he saw globules of fat circumscribed, red and pretty like grains of red coral. This description seems to intimate the red globules, and it was only the 15th of August 1673, that Lewenhoeck took notice of the red globules of the blood. Transf. Philos. N° 102.

(*b*) One may suppose it is the opinion of Quesnai by what he saith. Œconom. Anim. Tom. III. p. 36. See what the celebrated Senac saith thereupon, in his Traité du Cœur, tom. II. p. 662.

on the re-union of a great number of globules, I having often obferved, in the fmalleft veffel, folitary fingle globules very red, moving in a row, and at the fame time a collection of a great number in the large veffels, appearing yellow and even pale (c).

The fize of thefe globules is very fmall, for, on obferving with the fame folar microfcope one globule, and a little feather of the wing of a butterfly, the globule appeared to me at leaft one thoufand times fmaller; and I fhould be very much inclined to admit the Englifh calculations, which make 1940 (d) or even 3240 diameters of a globule to make an inch: and I think this too low a calculation. On examining them with a glafs, magnifying the diameter of the object 250 times, their diameter hath not appeared to me larger than the twentieth part of an inch, which gives, with refpect to this diameter, to an inch 1,5000.

There hath been lately fome doubt with refpect to their figure, whether they were fpherical, or whether their different diameters were unequal Lewenhoeck (f) and G.

(c) Thefe are the veffels, in which M de Sauvage faith are only found yellow globules Pulfus Theor p 24
(d) Jurin Philof Tranfac N° 377, art 7
(e) Hale's Hæmaftat p 56 in his remarks
(f) Experim & Contem T. II p 73 & feq

W.

W. Muys (*g*) have obferved, that thofe of fifh and of other animals that have cold blood, were flat and at the fame time oval, fo that each globule had three different diameters; the greateft is that of its length, the magnitude makes the mean diameter, and the thicknefs makes the fmalleft. M. Miles (*h*) and M. Senac, (*i*) have in general given them the figure and form of a lentile; this laft efpecially faith, they are eliptic and flat in frogs: he imagines even to have obferved an edge almoft tranfparent in their circumference.

I have often examined them, and particularly the half circumferences of the globules, which feem to form a fmall eminence upon the membranes of the veins; they appeared to me thick in frogs, and obferving the variations that were produced by different rays of light, the diameter of the thicknefs appeared to me to be equal to that of the length, or at leaft very near the matter, the diameter of the magnitude did not feem to be lefs. It is very difficult to give any pofitive opinion of any object fo fmall and fo moveable, what I can fay with certainty is, that always when I faw globules extravafated between the membranes of the Myfentery,

(*g*) Fabric Mufculor, p 300. & feq
(*h*) Tranfac Philof N? 460, p 726.
(*i*) L c p 656.

I never could observe one diameter greater than another, but I am in some doubt whether my eye hath deceived me. Those who have made use of the solar microscope, have also observed the spheric Moleculæ, although this instrument renders the Peripheries less distinct than the ordinary microscopes. Mr Baker, on observing these globules with this microscope, compares them to grains of pepper (*k*).

But you will ask, if they change their figure? Many authors of credit long ago have reported (*l*), that the compression which the globules undergo in passing into the extremities of the smaller vessels, changeth their figure; that the diameters become unequal, the longest being that which is parallel to the axis, and the shortest that which is parallel to the diameter of the vessels. I do not deny my having seen something of this nature, especially when the globules pass through curves and flexions of the small vessels, but I do not care to assert this as an absolute truth.

(*k*) Philof Transac N° 458, p 517

(*l*) Lewenhoeck Exper Contem p 61, and in other places, James Keill of muscular motion, p 163, H Miles Philosoph Transac N° 460, M Senac Traite du Cœur, l 2 p 657 The celebrated Van Swieten, saith he hath observed it in the pulmonary vessels of water lizards Comment in Aphoris Boerhaave, Tom I p 145, F W Horch Miscel Ptrochurs. Tom. VI p 116, and many other authors.

I find the late Mr. Platner *(m)* too positive, and all who like him have denied these globules, or have taken them for adipose or fatty masses, since they are certainly distinct circumscribed Moleculæ, of a different nature from the other humours, always like themselves, and intirely independent of any accidental formation.

Whatever some authors *(n)* have imagined of them, it will be found very improbable that they contain air, if one does but consider their solidity, which is sensible to the eye, and what we know in other respects, that the red part of the blood is the heaviest *(o)*, and sinks to the bottom of the serosity *(p)*. and indeed one could not think otherwise of those globules that contain some particles of iron, whose specific gravity is to that of the serosity, as 7 to 1. Another proof that they contain no air is, that when a candle is brought near the Mesentery of a frog, so as to

(m) Differt. de Noxis cohibit. Suppurat. N° 6 Hartsoeker Eſſaits p 5

(n) Bohn Circ p 179 George Cheyne's Philosophical principles of Religion, p 304 G Erchard Hamberger Physiolog Medic p 16, 17 T Knight's vindication, p 4 and some others

(o) Jurin Differt 8 p 99, gives the proportion of the weight of the red globules to that of the serosity, as 1054, 1030, and the celebrated M. Thomas Schwenke as 1240, 1142, Hæmatolog p 123

(p) Morgan's Philosophic Princip p 114, saith a drop of blood falling into water disengageth itself of its fat, and sinks to the bottom

heat the blood, even almost so near as to burn it. The globules, do not at all dilate themselves, which they would consequenly do if they contained air neither do they at all dilate themselves in the receiver of an air-pump *(q)*, when the air is drawn off. From hence we learn what we ought to think of any hypothesis, founded on a supposition, that the globules are bullæ full of air

I have observed many changes these globules undergo The first, which happens very easily, is their coagulation, this is formed from clots of blood, by the re-union of eight or a greater number of globules, which very often shuts up the passage of the blood in the vessels, especially in the places where there happens to be Aneurisms or Varices, yet the strength of the heart prevailing, propels these grumous parts, and thereby makes the passages free · this happens in large Aneurisms I have seen one in the neck of a very great magnitude, filling all the carotid artery, I found this Aneurisme filled with a thick and grumous blood Some celebrated writers have taken notice of this before me *(r)*, and Lewenhoeck *(s)* hath observed this in frogs.

(q) Juin D. Tert p 100
(r) With respect to the Varices, M de Sundrie de Natura Sanguinis, p 218 With respect to the Aneurisms, the Memoirs of the royal Academy of Sciences, anno 1707, p 21
, Experim & Contemp p 179

The second change the red globules undergo, is when they lose their motion in the veins; they then seem to be changed into oil, and afterwards into a kind of ointment, wherein one may observe a few striæ or lines, like what is observed in distilling oils. but in the great number of experiments which I have made on frogs, I never found that they formed themselves into polygon plexuses like network. This change, however, doth not destroy the nature of the globules, for bleeding or heat destroy this unctuosity, and establisheth a distinction between each globule: but when the globules are strayed out of their vessels, either arterial or venal, not only in animals that have warm blood, but also in frogs, they become grumous.

Another considerable change of the blood, is the formation of the lumps and clots that shut up wounded vessels. I intend to speak of this, after I have said something concerning the transparent part of the blood, of which one can have no idea by observing the vessels in a state of plenitude. For in the arteries and veins of a frog in health and well fed, the red globules seem so entirely to fill them, that one would not imagine they could contain any thing besides. M. V Menghini (*t*) believed there was proportionally fewer red globules in frogs than in men; but I cannot

(*t*) Commentar. Acad Bonon T. 2. p 2 p 238

conceive how one could add more of these red globules to the vessels, since they already so fill the canals as to prevent a discovery of any one transparent point; and M. Pujati (u) is much in the right in saying, that the transparent serosity, in which the globules swim, is not to be perceived.

But notwithstanding this impossibility of seeing in some cases this fluid, it is easy to demonstrate as to the small vessels, that they contain a very fine and thin fluid. It is sufficient for that purpose, to observe the considerable intervals that appear in a row of these globules, which are often found distant from one another, and yet are in continual motion. This seems an evident proof, that there is between these separated globules, a fluid which serves to impart from the one to the other, even to those of the extremities, the most distant from the heart, a motion which they impress to those that are in immediate contact with them: moreover we see very frequently in large arteries, spaces that appear empty, and in which the red globules possess but a very small part of the cavity of the vessel. One may suppose, that this apparent empty space must necessarily be filled with some transparent liquor. How can it happen that membraneous vessels, such as the arteries and veins should remain in a state of dilation,

(u) De Morbo Naronenf, p. 104.

if they were not full? I have often observed red globules drawn towards the cavity of an Aneurisme, and which were repulsed from the same, before they had touched any red blood, a demonstrative proof that they had met some other fluid, which was to me invisible, and which had resisted them. But the existence of this transparent fluid, shews itself more evidently yet, when an artery or vein is opened by bleeding, (for after the first force of the blood is over, and it bleeds but slowly, one may observe a kind of cloud to surround the wound or orifice, composed of a liquor that by degrees becomes white, and which changeth itself into a tumour, which one would think was formed by the very membranes of the vessel, and in the middle of which one may discover a red point, which is exactly situate on the orifice of the vessel) one may observe presently afterwards that the wound closes itself again under this tumour, and the blood retakes its natural course in the vessel. It cannot be denied, but that this cloud may be formed by a white fluid, since it hath been observed, that the globules extravasated between the membranes of the Mesentery or of the arteries, do not undergo the like change, but first form little distinct grumes, and afterwards the unctuosity and oily matter before taken notice of. herein is no cause of doubt, either

either with respect to the red grume which closeth large wounds (*w*), nor with respect to this white concretion last mentioned (*x*), which gives rise to polypuses, and to those white laminæ found so often in Aneurisms, and which I have observed to invest the internal membrane of the carotid and jugular (*y*).

But I have not been able to distinguish the parts which constitute this white fluid, even with microscopes that magnify much more than those of Leewenhoeck, and I can hardly believe, that it is possible to discover any yellow globules smaller than the red ones. neither do I think it is possible to be certain, that they are parts of the red globules, and that by their re-union they can again become globules of this colour. This hath created some arguments very plausible (*z*)

(*x*) Andrew Pasta De motu Sanguinis post ortum ed. t. 2. N° 75. Pet. Memoirs of acad. royal of scien. 1732, p. 304, and 1735, p. 442. M. Morand ibid. 1736. M. Monard Med. Ess. of the Soc. of Edin. t. 2. p. 273. Mem. of Chirurg. t. 2. p. 537, 542, 544, 117.

( ) M. Remus, in the dissert. before cited. M. Senac t. 2. p. 62, 260.

(*y*) I have given this observation in the introduction of the dispute of M. G. Zinn, and in the Pathologic. works. There is an account in the Memoirs of the Acad. Royal of Sciences 1732, p. 393, of a false Aneurisme, in which was found a mass formed of lamellæ, produced from thickened lympn.

(*z*) Lewenhoeck speaks of en of globules smaller than the red ones. Experim. & Contemp. p. 2, 3, 12, 15, 50, after him Boerhave and almost all the physiologists, have built on this foundation.

But

But it is impossible to ground this opinion on observation, since thereby there is not any one globule observed smaller than those of the red class, neither does observation teach us any thing concerning their resolution into smaller globules. The celebrated M. Senac (*a*) is of my opinion, which I think an honour

I have never yet observed any fat in the blood of frogs, and I suspect very much that what Malpighy thought was fat, was only bullæ of air, like those I have often observed circulating in the blood-vessels with great rapidity, and what Rodi (*b*) and Caldesi (*c*) had observed in the veins of frogs.

I do not conclude from this experiment, that there is air in the vessels of an animal in health; for in fifty experiments, there will be found only one that shall shew these bullæ of air, and only then when some wound hath

---

(*a*) Traité du Cœur, t 2 p 91, 660, he believes the cause of this error is, because when one red globule is observed alone, it appears sometimes yellow. The coagulum, which is formed by globules, when at rest, may have given room for some idea of their composition, by the re-union of globules of an inferior order, and the opinion that supposeth the yellow globules, formed from the resolution of the red ones, ariseth from the dissolution of this coagulum, produced either by heat or putrefaction

(*b*) Epistol ad Stenon This letter may be found in the supplement to Giorn de Litterati, tom III p 86

(*c*) Observ anat. intorno alle Tartarughe, p 67

happened to some large vessel, by which the air introduced itself. They are one thousand times at least larger than the blood-globules, and it is impossible therefore, that they should pass into the small vessels of one globule diameter. I have not discovered filaments in the blood, and it would be impossible, that long flexile bodies should, through so narrow a base, receive a motion sufficient to overcome the resistances of the small vessels (d).

What I have further to add is, that I have never been able to see distinctly the globules of animals that have warm blood. If after the manner of Lewenhoeck and Antony Hude, you put your blood into a capillary tube, the parieties of the tube, in adapting the microscope, creates so much obscurity, that it is impossible to distinguish any thing (e). If you extend a mouse like a frog under Lieburkuhn's microscope, the opacity of the coats of the Mesentery irrely conceals the vessels, and the laying bare the vessels produceth a coagulum of the blood by the cold air. one can only observe branches like coral.

No difference is found in the arterial and venal blood of frogs both equally condenseth itself into red grumes, but in a dog and in other animals that have warm blood, I have

(d) See M. Senac's reasons, tom II p 103, 104
(e) You find the same experiment in the differt of M. Remus, p. 39

experienced

experienced one hundred times that there was no difference, with respect to the colour or disposition, to coagulate between the blood of the artery and the pulmonary vein: but in some singular experiments made on a dog and a great rat, I have observed the artery and crural vein to give blood of a different colour; the first had very red blood and the vein very black. This difference of colour is not to be attributed to the action of the lungs. I have seen a much more remarkable difference in the vein of a frog, it was filled with two streams of blood of different colours; the column which came from the heart was purple, and that which returned from the side of the Intestines was of a pale yellow colour: and in general, whatever may be the action of the heart and lungs on the blood, the rapidity with which it circulates in the vessels, and the little time it is in the lungs, and the extreme small time there must be for the blood which was a little before venal to become arterial, prove that there must be but very little difference between the arterial blood from the pulmonary vein, and the venal blood from the Cava (*f*), and as both this blood contains the same globules, their difference can only consist in the proportion

(*f*) It is a long while since a man born for observations, the immortal Harvey, thought no credit was to be given to this difference.

of these globules with the limpid fluid, or in the nature of this fluid itself. but the white fluids escape our sight, and the experiments that have been made to decide the proportion of globules, to the serum in both this blood, do not agree among themselves (g). It is seldom that milk and chyle appear in the blood, I have nevertheless distinctly observed a very white chyle running into the axillary vein and I have attentively observed the right auricle, at each contraction, to propel a white liquor into the heart.

CHAP. III.

On the Motion of the Arterial Blood.

THE first motive that determined me thoroughly to examine this matter, was the opinions warranted almost by all the physiologists contrary to my experiments. The discoveries which I have made by the opening of a great number of

(g) Many authors believe the arterial blood more dense, and among others M. de Sauvage, de Inflamat p. 244. Others find more water in the arteries and their blood therefore more fluid. M. Ramnarschmid my pupil, hath found it lighter than very modern experiments. This variety in observations serve to prove, that if there is any difference in this respect, it is very inconsiderable

living and dead animals, are so different from what is generally shewed at any university, that I do not expect to see them established, until other anatomists have repeated the same; and indeed that must be done very often, in order to be acquainted with nature, and to learn to distinguish what is usual and constant, from what is extraordinary and accidental. Always when I observed any phænomenon which seemed to me of any importance, and which destroyed any part of the received theories, I have repeated the same experiment twenty times and oftner, until I was convinced of the certitude and constancy of the phænomenon, taking great care not to declare a fact for truth, whereof I had the least cause to doubt, For the sake of order in this dissertation, I intend to begin with the course of the arterial blood The concurrence of sentiments concerning the existence of its motion, from the heart even to the extremities, would be sufficient to confirm me that I am in no error by admitting the same: I have neverthelefs added to this testimony that of experiments, and have made all that could be endeavoured, as much as if Harvey and Wallæus had made none. Being persuaded that from hence we should receive a double advantage; repeated experiments give new force to what great men have taught us, and I hope to discover some truths that have
escaped

escaped them. This expectation is formed on that good intention nature hath been so kind to furnish me with, she is never consulted in vain, and always makes ample amends for the pains they undergo who study her. I will begin with the motion of the blood, because it may be observed without opening the vessels.

First, I am assured that the blood, propelled by the heart, dilates the arteries and creates what is called the pulse: this phænomenon sometimes is wanting in animals that have warm blood, perhaps because the coldness of the external air, coagulates the blood in the vessels. It hath been denied, that a pulse hath been observed on the opening of living animals (a), I have nevertheless very often seen in cats, dogs, and sheep, the pulsation of the arteries, they extend and sensibly affect the finger, on touching them at the time the heart contracts, if they are tied up their resilition not only becomes more sensible, but they appear to lengthen themselves, especially on observing them attentively at the angle of any flexion, wherein is very distinctly seen, even where there are no ligatures, that the part of the artery the nearest to the heart, lengthens itself, thereby making with the other branch, a more acute

---

(a) M. Sæhelin Dissert. de Pulsu, p. 9 teacheth us there was at Montpellier, a living dog without any sensible pulse

angle (*b*). The conical form of the arteries much contribute to the producing of this phænomenon, for it is for this reason, that the impulse of the blood, against the parieties of the arteries, is (in proportion to the distance) so much the greater, as they are the more distant from the heart. Experiments made upon the arteries, and even upon very small ramifications, as the Mammary, and others, have satisfied me, that they beat all at the same time, as also the coronary artery: although great men have told us, that this little artery is different from the others in this respect; but having opened it at different times, I always found that it spurts at the time of the heart's contraction, and that the blood runs slowly at the time of its relaxation (*c*).

The pulsation of the arteries become insensible, when they are of but one sixth part of a line diameter, I have observed it upon the membranes of the Intestines of a live animal, at the last curvature of an artery, and in the superior branch at the angles, but in the part of the artery beyond it was lost.

(*b*) M. Weitbrecht Comment. Acad. Petrop. tom. VII. p. 317, saith that all the artery is changed and displaced, and the celebrated M. Van Swieten hath observed the little arteries of a finger almost taken off, to lengthen themselves at every pulsation.

(*c*) M. Starle, p. 26 relates the same experiment in his excellent dissertation, De Reliquis Instrumentis quibus Sanguis in Circulum, &c N° 22.

The

The author, who hath lately afferted (*d*) that an artery, so far from dilating itself, contracts at the time of the pulsation, will be convinced, by taking an example from the heart and the Penis, that a fluid propelled in a flexile canal, may render it longer and larger at the same time.

I have found the number of pulsations in a fixed time, much more frequent than is commonly supposed, in taking an account, whereof I have more than once mitigated the anxiety which my indispositions had produced. I have observed that in a morning, after the warmth occasioned by being in bed was removed, my pulse was a little less frequent than at night, the number of pulsations in a minute was from 70 to 80 and this number is proportionally lessened, as a person is the less inclined to a fever, for in hypocondriacal cases, with watchings and sweating whole nights, the number of pulsations was only from 66 to 68. In general, in a phlegmatic person, we reckon 60 pulsations a minute, in a lively person from 68 to 80; after a meal, the number is in-

---

(*d*) Otia Physiologica, p. 26, he hath only renewed the opinion of James Primrose, the first adversary of the circulation, who wrote positively that at the time of the systole, the artery became more elevated and narrower. He gives, at the same time, a figure of this change, according to his imagination. De Struct. Fundamentor Plempii. 87.

creased

creased by 10 or 12 pulsations a minute. Hence it is, that those who are on the recovery from a dangerous illness, having often 90 pulsations in a minute, the increase which a meal procureth, raiseth the number to 100 and 108, which is a feverish state: when the time of sleep comes on, the number of pulsations increase even to 80 and 84 (e). This is doubtless one of the causes of the increase of fevers at night, for 10 pulsations added to 110, which is often observed in an ordinary fever, make 120, which would produce a fever that could not be long endured.

In fevers that intermit, on the days of intermission, there are generally observed 94 pulsations, and if there is somewhat of a fever 100; catarrhal fevers of the mildest sort, have 110 and 118 to 120. In the increase of a Quotidian, there is generally observed 114, and in a violent eresipelatous or miliary fevers, or in the paroxysm of a Tertian, this number is increased to 130 or 134. Above this number it is almost impossible to distinguish, and there is only to be perceived a continual fluttering. The paroxysm is always over, when there is observed not above 90 pulsations, and the danger of an acute fever is over, when the pulsations do not exceed that number. We

(e) Schwencke, p 140.

cannot form any judgment of heat or sweat by the pulse, I have been in a sweat without sleeping, with 66 pulsations, I was very drouthy with 134, with the same number of 66, I have had a moderate heat without any sweat, and with 100, to which the fever was reduced, I found myself well, and as a person that is neither hot nor cold. I have observed these same variations in a woman, of a constitution and age different from mine.

Give me leave to add the following phænomena concerning the pulse: if a ligature is made on the artery, the pulse ceaseth in the part of the artery that is under the ligature. Fallopius made this experiment, and made use of it to prove, against the doctrine of the schools, that the pulse did not depend on any force belonging to the artery (*f*). An Aneurisme, in this respect, does not produce the effect of a ligature. I have often observed, in artificial Aneurisms in frogs, that the motion of the blood appeared in reality slower in the tumour itself, yet the pulse had its natural frequency under the Aneurisme: this I have found by experiments on frogs. Harvey observed the pulse under the Aneurisme, but he said it was more feeble (*g*). Modern physicians say, that the pulse is produced by a wave of blood going

(*f*) De partibus Similaribus, p. 100.
(*g*) Dissertat. de Circulo Sanguinis, tom II p 215

out of the heart, with more swiftness than that which preceded, and had lost its force by the resistance of the small vessels; and that the resistance which this wave makes (*h*) against that which succeeds, is the cause that its direct course is impeded, and that a part of its force is exerted laterally against the parieties of the vessels, and elevates them.

What persuades me that the conical form is not the principal cause of the pulse, is, that the pulsations appear sensible, and are even very strong in the Carotids, which are not sensibly conical, and also are perceived in the very small cylindrical vessels. In frogs this force of the arterial blood, which produceth the systole of the heart (*i*), is not sensible, even by the microscope, while the animal preserves its strength: but it is observed

(*h*) M. De Sauvage de Pulsu, p. 19. and his Comment. on M. Hales's Hæmastaticks, p. 279.

(*i*) Antony De Heide de Ven. Section Experiment. p. 6. Henry Baker's Microscope made easy, p. 136, and George Adams p. 45, have observed this acceleration. Lewenhoeck's Experiment. & Contemp. p. 167, hath denied that it was perceived in the small vessels, and the theory of Bryan Robinson tends to the same negative opinion, Anim Œconom Propos 11. It is easy to account for these two different sentiments, by a very natural supposition, which is, that these observations were made at different times, Lewenhoeck made his observation when the animal was in full vigour, and the others when the strength was exhausted. What confirms me in this idea, is that Lewenhoeck himself has described this phænomenon in another place. Experim. & Cont. t. II. p. 175 & t. III. p. 114.

when the animal begins to grow weak, at which time we may distinctly perceive, that a fresh wave that comes from the heart, propels and drives forward that which preceded. The eye which cannot perceive the difference of 1001 and 1000, may distinguish very well the difference of 11 and 10, although both the one and other differ only in 1: after the pulsation, the artery remains equally full, and although its diameter decreaseth, yet it appears not to empty itself.

It is not sufficient for the formation of the pulse, that the heart drives the blood into the artery, but the artery must be capable of extension, so as to give way to this pressure: if it is too strong, the motion of the blood will take place, but it will be exactly as in a glass tube, and without any elevation of the parieties. In frogs the Aorta, the pulmonary artery, and the great vessels of the arm, have manifest pulsations; but the descending Aorta and largest trunks of the Mesentery have none, for their membranes are too strong, and it is impossible they should give way to the impulse, which the heart can impart to the blood: this I have seen one thousand times, and I may at any time (*k*)

(*i*) M. De Sauvage Pulſ. Theor. p. 24. to the truth of these experiments, and my pupil M. Remus p. 48, have reported this want of pulse in frogs, perhaps after my observations.

make

make the same observation with the same result. I have very often seen a vein so to lie on an artery, as to divide its smallest motions, yet it was not at all moved at the pulsation of the artery. Arteries that are ossified, have no pulsation (*l*), and nature hath been very prudent in preventing the arteries of frogs, which do not contract themselves, from being susceptible of dilation.

A second law of the motion of the blood in the arteries, which may be observed without opening them, is, that it is carried from the heart to all the extremities: this is proved by ligatures I have repeated Dr Harvey's experiments, I have put ligatures on the greater part of the arteries, and first on the Aorta, which I have very frequently tied at a small distance from its going off from the heart, in eels, frogs, dogs, cats, and other animals. It is astonishing to observe how much it swells between the ligature and the heart, it becomes of a brilliant red colour, and sensibly lengthens itself at each pulsation, during which time the heart is violently agitated by the continual irritation of the blood, whereof it endeavours in vain to discharge itself, this ligature is one of the causes which sustains the motion of the left ventricle, very long after that of the right is lost, which I have fully spoken of elsewhere (*m*). When the

(*l*) M Senac, tom II. p. 225.
(*m*) Commentar. Societ. Regiæ Gotting tom. I. p. 263 This memoir is reprinted and follows this.

artery under the ligature is touched, no pulsation is observed, and when it is opened, gives no blood (*n*).

I afterwards put a ligature on the pulmonary artery, which is not done without much difficulty, when I observed the same phænomena as before on tying up the Aorta, the right ventrical extremely full and extremely agitated, and the pulmonary artery excessively swelled, emitted its blood on being opened, with as much force as the Aorta itself. These experiments agree but little with what a certain geometrical physician advanceth more than once (*o*), which is, that ligatures make the arteries swell less than the veins, and that the swelling of the arteries, produced by ligatures, is almost insensible; yet it is certain that the Aorta of a frog, which is not larger than one of the small arteries of the human body, which anatomists hardly take any notice of, swells prodigiously when it is tied up or compressed, and that the experiment may succeed, as M. de Sauvage hath described it. The ligature must be made upon an artery, that its trunk may discharge itself into some branch above this ligature; and the ligature must be made only on very small arteries: if for example, ligatures are made on the mesenteric arteries of a frog,

(*n*) Drelincourt Canicid 1.
(*o*) Theoria Tumor. p. 19. Pulsus Theor. p. 26

which are only capillary veſſels in a dog the blood immediately becomes immoveable in that branch that is tied up, without any ſwelling, preſently after it becomes retrogade in the neighbouring ramifications, and leaves its veſſel intirely empty even to the ligature, and filled underneath by the blood that was there, whoſe motion the ligature had ſtopped. This ſingular fact ſeems to depend (*p*) on the hardneſs of the artery, which the force of the heart in this animal could not overcome; and on the motion of attraction, of which I ſhall ſpeak in another place; and alſo on the facility that the blood finds in paſſing from one branch to another. I muſt moreover remark with M de Sauvage, that the blood doth not always make ſuch efforts againſt the obſtructed veſſels, as ſome phyſiologiſts have imagined (*q*), but it paſſeth inſenſibly and eaſily into the neighbouring veſſels, which it dilates ſucceſſively. hence the veſſels of the Pelvis become very large, after a ligature is made on the umbilical arteries.

When a ligature is made on an artery in animals which have warm blood, a conſiderable tumour forms itſelf above the ligature,

(*p*) M Remus hath been a witneſs of this as well as myſelf, p 49, 50.

(*q*) Cheſelden before cited p. 203 Hoffman de Elaſticit Fibra p 9, 10, where he reports an experiment on frogs which makes againſt him, the celebrated M. Senac, t II p 172.

which neverthelefs diminifheth gradatim, although the ligature remains on, which afterwards becomes changed into a ligament, whofe internal furface is filled with a filamentous white fubftance: the fame happens in the umbilical arteries. In arteries that are obftructed, even in the Carotid, according to Mr Emet's experiment (*r*). I cannot fee by all thefe facts, how M. de Sauvage could conclude, that a ligature creates a lefs tumour in the arteries than in the veins, for the experiment on the Aorta of frogs, which I have abovementioned, fufficiently proves the contrary, and the fwiftnefs of the arterial blood was a fufficient proof at firft fight, and the more fo, becaufe the veins have a greater number of ramifications for receiving their blood

I now return to my experiments When a ligature is made on an artery in the lower belly, it fwells and hath a pulfation above the ligature; it emptieth itfelf alfo above, and when it is opened in this place, it emits no blood: the animal, as Steno hath already obferved, loofeth the motion of his legs, cannot ftand on his feet, and moves them after him, as if he dragged fome heavy weight I have fometimes obferved convulfions in thefe parts, I have repeated, and mention here this experiment, becaufe it had been doubted by

(*r*) Teutamen 2 p. 27

great men (s): it does not succeed in frogs; and although the Aorta is tied up or divided, they can leap and make their escape. A ligature on the thoracic Aorta, produceth in a cat the most violent symptoms, the whole animal becomes stupid and insensible. When a ligature is made on the Carotid in live animals, or the mesenterick artery, or the Crurale or Brachial, every where the same phænomena appear. A tumour above the ligature, which the congestion of blood renders of a shining colour, there is a pulsation, and the artery lengthens itself at the time of the systole of the heart, and diminisheth in the Diastole, the motion of the legs or the other members, undergo no alteration (t), and a ligature, even on the Carotid, hath not created any considerable change. What I have hitherto related may be sufficient to teach us, that the blood passeth from the heart into the Aorta, and from the Aorta into all the arteries of the whole body. I must at present speak of those motions of the blood that are less apparent, and which are made in a more obscure manner, and also which are not perceived until the vessels are opened, unless their membranes are transparent, as they generally are in frogs. On

(s) Swammerdam Biblia Nat p. 850, and author of a new memoir on the motion of the muscles, presented to the academy of Berlin, N° 20.

(t) Drelincourt Canicid 9

these animals chiefly and on fish, I have observed these motions, and will now set forth exactly what appeared to me.

The first phænomenon that offers itself, is the rapidity with which the globules of blood move from the heart to the extremities, as I have observed it in the Mesentery of a frog, in the membranes for the spawn, and in the tails of fish: it is very difficult to establish any proportion between the space it had passed, and the time employed in passing, because the space that is circumscribed by a microscope is so small, that the time which the blood must employ in passing, is less than any sensible measure. The inequality of swiftness in the motion of the blood in animals that have cold blood, seems to be the reason that persuaded Dr. Hales (*u*), that its motion was forty-three times more swift in the lungs of a frog, than in the muscles As for my part, I have not observed that it moved in the lungs with any greater velocity, than in the Mesentery; but I have very distinctly seen, that it had less velocity by far, than the blood that spurts from an artery that is opened. I cannot see what should occasion this very great swiftness in the lungs of frogs. it is true, that at first sight we very distinctly see in these animals, that at the time when the lungs are expanded, their principal artery,

u Hæmerstat p 68

which

which extends itfelf their whole length, and which ramifies from one part to another, becomes almoft ftraight, and makes a very eafy paffage for the blood, but at the time when this vifcus fubfides, as in expiration, the artery is found contorted in a ferpentine manner, making the paffage for the blood more difficult. But this particular quality of the lungs, is no proof againft the velocity of the blood in other parts, in which it, at all times, finds the fame eafe for its circulation: moreover it frequently happens, that the blood circulates with a much greater velocity in an artery of the Mefentery, when it moves very flow, or is even intirely at reft in the others Hence we may obferve, there is nothing extraordinary in thofe topical fevers and heat incident to any limb: I have moreover obferved, that the blood was much lefs retarded in the fmall veffels, than the geometrical phyficians imagine. In frogs it is impoffible to diftinguifh any difference between the velocity that is obferved in the ramifications of the arteries, and that which is obferved in the trunks, and it feems to have the fame velocity in the largeft mefenteric veffels, as in its laft vifible fubdivifion I have feen in a dog, which is an animal that hath warm blood, this fluid to fpring from a fmall ramification of the mammaries, of lefs than half a line diameter, to the

the distance of six feet and an half; and that in another dog, of which *Keill* opened the Iliac artery, it sprung not above one half of this distance (*x*) There is also a much greater velocity in the small vessels of fish, as I shall prove by an experiment, which I shall relate in speaking of the veins.

If the velocity of the blood in frogs was the same as in man, according to *Keill's* calculations (*y*), which are, that in the vessels of one globule diameter, it should go in a minute only the $\frac{1}{1425}$ of an English foot, but I have often seen, in the small mesenteric vessels of a frog, that the velocity was so great, that I could hardly follow it with my eye, and that sometimes it equalled, and at other times exceeded that of the blood in the great vessels, although, according to these calculations, it should have been 1448 times slower (*z*). But if this velocity is so considerable in the small veins, it must be more so in the small arteries from which these veins have their origin and motion, and more considerable yet in the arteries that are larger than the capillary ones I have even seen veins, of one or two globules diameter, to carry their blood with a sufficient velocity, though in the large arteries it was very small; and indeed

(*x*) De Vi Cordis, p. 41 t I. fol 5 the Holland edit
(*y*) De Velocitate Sanguinis, p 36.
(*z*) De Secretiore Animal, p 56, the same edition

what the more takes away all cause for doubts is, that in observing a branch which arose from a trunk much larger, and which returned up again the length of this same trunk, I observed that the blood had a much greater velocity in the branch than in the trunk. I have not had in view, in repeating these experiments, any intention of publishing what errors there may be in the calculations of great men, who have treated of these matters; I only set out honestly facts, which are proofs very superior to theories, and which shew us, that the velocity is very great in the small vessels, other experiments establish the velocity, by which the perspiring vessels emit their vapour. Accurate observations will prove the truth of what I am going to relate, concerning the motion of the arterial blood The red globules swim equally distributed in the serosity without any confusion, and are moved in right parallel lines, without rubbing or mixing themselves together, and without any manner of rotation (*a*); so that all that hath been reported concerning the vortical confused motions of the blood, hath no manner of foundation, with respect to animals that have cold blood, for the experiments which I have made, in order to observe its motion in those animals that have warm blood, have not succeeded. The pressure of

(*a*) G. E. Remus, p 37, 43, &c

the

the blood against the parieties of the vessels, and against the resistances it meets with at the divisions of the arteries, is not very great, it is easy without any repulsion, and it is very far from dividing and resolving the globules, or changing their figure and it is so easy, that it discomposeth not the weak covering of the air which forms the bullæ, which are frequently seen in the vessels of frogs. when the progressive motion of the blood is stopped, the globules become immoveable, and remain always at rest until the cause is removed. Hence we see that eminent men (b), who have supposed in the blood an intestinal motion, capable of contributing to its progressive motion, are quite deceived. I have repeated this experiment so often and with such constant success, that I am persuaded nothing can ever be alledged against me, I have often carefully observed if I could perceive any difference between the velocity of different globules in the same artery. it seemed to me, that those which were in the center, and which moved in the Axis of the vessel, have a greater velocity than those which touch the parieties, and this observation is consonant to those of Malpighy (c) and Schreiber (d)

(b) B Stevenson in the Essays of Edinburg, tom. V p 2
(c) Posthum p 92
(d) Elementa Medic p 323

When

When an artery divides itself, the globules, if there is no disorder in the circulation, divide themselves proportionally between the two branches, and I have carefully observed, if in the angles of the vessels, there was any difference in the velocity of the blood in coming to these angles. I have observed in frogs, different branches arising from trunks under different angles, and when I found no natural angles and curves, I made some. This is the result, such as I find by experiments; for I have not repeated them often enough to be assured, that nothing remains for discovery on this article, this observation being attended with much difficulty.

The first artery that I observed, divided itself into four branches; two went off from the trunk in a right angle, the two others separated a little from the direction of the superior trunk, with which they formed very acute angles. I observed for near six hours, that the branches which went off in a right angle, discontinued their motion much sooner than the two others, a second artery divided itself in a different manner, the more considerable branch went off but little from the direction of the trunk; the other much smaller formed a considerable angle with the trunk. I could not immediately distinguish any difference in the velocity in either of these vessels; but when the motion of the blood began to abate,

abate, I obferved that it continued much longer in thofe branches that went off in the leaft angle from the direction of the trunk. It appears by this obfervation, that the velocity in the branches is fo much the greater, the lefs the angle is they make with the trunk, and this is found confonant to the theory of M M de Sauvage (*e*), Senac (*f*), and Hales (*g*). M. Remus (*h*), hath made thefe experiments with me. The event is not always the fame, and I have often obferved the motion to ceafe in an artery, and yet continue in a branch that went off from it in a right angle.

I much defired to know what was in a living animal, the effect of curvatures in the veffels, I knew very well, that they have much influence on the injections that are made on a dead fubject, and that it is fufficient to bring back an arm upon the body, whereby an angle is made at the fubclavian artery, that the injection may fail in this member, becaufe of the difficulty that it finds in entering it. In order to fatisfy myfelf on this article, I detached an artery from its cellular membrane that connected it to the Mefentery,

(*e*) Differtation fur les medicaments qui affectent certaines parties du corps, p 26

(*f*) Tom II p 167

(*g*) Hæmaftaticks, p 67, hath given experiments her upon

(*h*) Page 43

and turned it side-ways, so as to make it form a considerable curve. but I could not observe, that the velocity of the blood was thereby diminished (1) I took another artery and turned it to a point, so that it made a very acute angle, with that part of the trunk that was the nearest the heart, but this flexion did not yet diminish the velocity of the blood, from whence I conclude, as I shall say presently, that the force of the heart is strong enough to overcome, without any sensible diminution of its power, any resistances of this kind: but I speak with respect only to simple flexions, and not of those which are so complex as in the Epididymis. The whole world agrees, that these much retard the course of the Semen · in order to be convinced thereof, we need only consider how slowly mercury passeth them, and also a little reflect how much force any fluid must lose in overcoming obstacles so long continued.

Lastly, in frequently observing first natural Aneurisms, and afterwards those which I created myself, I began distinctly to distinguish the change of motion in a fluid passing from a narrow canal into a vessel that is larger, like that which happens to the water of any river that dischargeth itself into a lake or pool. The velocity of the blood dimi-

---

(1) Theory made M. Micholotte thus judge of this matter, De Secret. Fluidor. p 139, 140.

nisheth sensibly in the cavities of Aneurisms, and circulates through them but slowly, which may give rise to a re-union of the globules, and a simple coagulum may be formed by the connection of many globules together, and which the force of the heart may resolve, by putting into motion the disunited globules. It will be more surprising to find, that under the Aneurisme, the blood resumes its former velocity, and moves with as much rapidity as before it entered the same, and though the blood moves very slowly in the Aneurisme, the propelling force, which seems almost exhausted in this part, is renewed, whereby the blood receives its natural velocity. It is not seldom that we observe the blood to move with a greater velocity in a ramification, than in the trunk from which it ariseth.

This experiment, which I have often repeated, seems to me very important, and in a manner radically disproves all that hath been asserted with so much gloss, concerning the pretended diminution of the velocity of the blood in the small vessels (*k*).

It seems that in animals the power of the heart is much superior to the resistance that

(*k*) Keill establisheth the Ratio between the velocity of the blood in the Aorta, and of that in the capilary vessels, as 5233 1 Robinson as 1100 1, Butler as 500 1, but the celebrated Dr Hales hath not taken notice, that the motion of the blood was very slow in the capillary vessels

can

can arise from the smallness of the vessels; and it always happens in that case, that the velocity is increased in canals, in proportion to the diminution of their diameter. We have an example hereof in fountains, whereof the water riseth with greater force the narrower their tubes are, as far as to the point where the force of adhesion, between the fluid and the parieties of the tube, becomes stronger than that of the impulsion, which is a case particular, and has nothing to do in this place.

The theoreme which I have now established, wants not much demonstration If the case was otherwise, the minuteness of the vessels would diminish the velocity of the fluids, if the force of the frictions produced a decreased velocity in proportion to the diminution of diameters, in that case it must happen, that the blood, in passing from an Aneurisme, or from any large vessel into another that is narrower, would diminish its velocity, but by observation we may observe the contrary, as I have before related. tI will perhaps be an objection to me, that I have in my observations made use of a microscope, which makes the velocity of the blood seem greater but this objection cannot avail, because I have used a microscope in observing the great trunks as well as the small vessels; therefore the increased velocity being the

same

same, similitudes are not changed, by which only, as to this matter, we are to form a judgment

I have been desirous to observe what happens in the Anastomosis's, and at the re-union of two vessels meeting by opposite directions I have found that in this case the two currents reciprocally resist each other, and that the globules of the one strike against those of the other, until the weaker current gives way and is overcome by the stronger · the same nearly happens with the blood flowing from an artery that is divided, and which generally runs by two opposite currents. If it flows from some branch of an Anastomosis, or from a flexion of an artery, it is to be presumed that the two currents will meet there, as the two currents of an artery that is wounded meet and flow out of the wound. From hence it may be concluded, that in the human body, where there are very frequent Anastomosis's, the blood may be moved in different directions, according as one of the branches, communicating with the other, shall have a greater or less velocity than its companion As for example, in the arteries that are found between the back and the palm of the hand, and which I have called perforantes superiores (*l*), it is evident, according to the situation of the hand, that the weight of the blood will determine its

(*l*) Iconum Anatomicarum Fascic 6 p 41, 42

course, either from the palm to the back of the hand, or from the back to the palm. I will set forth in another chapter the power of this weight, which will be found one of the causes of the motion of the blood.

It appears that the great design of nature, in thus multiplying the arterial circles and the Anastomosis's, hath been in a manner for this purpose: viz. if a trunk should be obstructed, destroyed, or obliterated, its branches may receive blood from the neighbourly trunks. This I have with satisfaction observed in human subjects, wherein I have found a carotid, a vertebral, or a brachial artery, obstructed, ossified, and useless, and yet the circulation not discomposed.

I must now speak of the irregularities that happen in the motion of the blood; sometimes it is retarded and troubled, sometimes it seems obstructed by somewhat it is endeavouring to overcome, sometimes it is retrograde, sometimes at rest, and the vessels become empty.

The retardation of the blood, is generally the first of all these irregularities.

The velocity is troubled when it is in general diminished, and all of a sudden a new effort of the heart renews the velocity, which in a moment after it looseth again (*m*). In-

(*m*) A Van Lewenhoeck hath observed somewhat like this. Experim. & Contemp. p. 159, 165, 179, &c. G. Adams, l. c. p. 45.

arition is generally joined to this flowness of motion, and generally few globules are observed in a vessel wherein this lentor predominates. Always when the motion of the blood recovers itself, after any diminution or retrogradation, we distinctly see every wave make a resistance to that which follows, and that this last must consequently impart to the other its natural motion. Hence we see, that this resistance, which one wave creates to another, ought to be taken notice of in the general resistance which the heart meets with, and it ought not to be neglected when we would make an estimation of it (*n*)

Oscillation is almost a constant effect of the retardation of the arterial motion, in this case the blood goes and comes, and alternately it pursues its natural course, and becomes afterwards retrograde (*o*)

This fluctuation is very singular in the places where the artery widens itself, sometimes the blood of one of the branches in its retrogradation, makes a resistance to the blood of the trunk, which being of superior force, repels it either into its own proper branch, or into some other, from whence it returns some little time after it had been at rest, to be

(*n*) Morron Lettres, p. 26
(*o*) This motion of Oscillation is described in Leuwenhoeck Experim & Contemp, 164, 165, 186, 188 tom III p 111, 112, and in Boerhaave De Usu ratiocinii Mechan p 34 see also F. W Horen L c p 115

repelled

repelled again as before (*p*): at other times one of the branches, capable of making a greater refiftance, forceth its blood to run back into another, either crofs the trunk, or upwards towards the heart by the fame trunk.

I have feen in a branch, which went off from the trunk under a very great angle, that the blood became retrograde with fo great a force, that after fome ofcillations, it re-eftablifhed the natural courfe of the blood, in the part of the trunk that was inferior to the rife of the branch. This produced a frefh ofcillation between the branch, and the fuperior trunk, in which there were but few globules, and the trunk by this ofcillation recovered its natural motion; fo that the trunk and the branch formed two fources, which conveyed the blood into the inferior trunk as into a common refervoir. This continued fome time; and this confufion terminated at laft, by the ceffation of the retrograde motion of the branch, and the fuperior trunk difcharged its blood into its two divifions, as in the natural ftate: but before this was compleated, there were obferved, defcending from the fuperior trunk, clouds formed by collections of the globules; and this obftacle having been overcome, all was reftored to their natural ftate. I have alfo obferved a remarkable ofcillation,

(*p*) M. Miles hath obferved the fame. See the Tranf. Phil. vol. 41. N°. 460. p. 728.

between the coagulated blood in an Aneurifme, and the blood of part of the artery which had yet preferved its motion, sometimes the globules of the Aneurifme gave way to the blood of the artery, and the next moment the globules repelled it, and forced it to pafs into other branches that made no refiftance. What is moft particular in this ofcillation is, that the globules of the arterial blood were repulfed by an invifible fluid, before they came into contact with the red blood of the Aneurifme. Thefe ofcillations, with which I have fo often entertained myfelf, terminate and end either by the re eftablifhment of a natural ftate (*q*), when the force and power of the heart begins to prevail, or by an intire retrogreffion or a ceffation of motion, which is known by the longer diftance of the intervals of thefe ofcillations.

It often happens, that the power of the heart re-eftablifhes the natural motion of the blood; and the refolution of the grumes of blood, produced by thefe ofcillations, difcover to us one of the advantages arifing from Anaftomofis's, which is to overcome obftructions arifing by the blood which an artery, void of any obftructions, propels againft that blood that is beginning to be at reft.

(*q*) A Lewenhoeck Experim & Contemp tom ii p 104, 165, tom iii p 112.

Retrocessions are pretty frequent, they are oftener seen in the veins or arteries after the heart is divided, and are observed, though the power of this muscle begins to diminish, and though the circulation begins to abate. At this time the blood of the branches or ramifications go back into the trunks, and from thence towards the heart, sometimes it happens, that its progressive motion is performed regularly in some branches, although in others it is retrograde: I have observed this both in fish as well as frogs. Very large vessels are subject to this irregularity, at a time when the motion was natural in the small ones; I have observed two branches of the same trunk, the one carried its blood forward, in the other it moved in a contrary direction, and was repelled from the branch into the trunk, I took notice, that commonly the cause of this retrocession, was some obstruction, as an Aneurisme, in which the coagulated blood makes a resistance to that coming from the arteries, and compels it to a retrogradation: this preternatural motion does not cease until the grumes of blood that occasioned it have been carried off. Lastly, retrogradations take place after large wounds, and especially after the amputation of the heart and in the arteries, wherein the motion of the blood ceaseth. M. Senac (r) hath taken no-

(r) Traité du Cœur, tom. ii. p. 174.

tice, that fainting is one of the causes of this retrogradation of the blood.

These frequent retrogradations deceived old Mr. Lewenhoeck, who was a diligent observer, yet a man of little learning; he confounded the veins with the arteries, and ascribed, many years before his death, the acceleration and pulsation (s), and also the blood's course towards the heart to the venal blood, and ascribed to the arteries its slowness, rest, and return towards this muscle.

The cessation of motion puts an end to all, and this cessation always remains in the arteries of frogs, when any artery hath discharged all its blood, or when it receives no more from the Aorta.

This case I have often seen in frogs, not only in those which had fasted a long while, but also in those that had been well fed; their arteries are sometimes found intirely empty, and seem like white nerves, with which indeed Lewenhoeck hath confounded them (t). This phænomenon perhaps is the cause that deceived the ancients, who imagined that the arteries contained only air: it is very certain that they are sometimes intirely empty, although eminent men

(s) Enstol Physiologic. tom IV. p. 167. Philosoph. Transact. N° 319. V. Uffenbach. Reisen, tom. III. p. 350.
(t) T. u Epistle 119. p. 112.

have

have been of another opinion; sometimes it happens that the blood is at rest in some branches, when it is in motion in others: that is to say the small vessels, for these preserve their motion after the trunks have lost theirs.

Also it frequently happens, that when the animal becomes languid, the blood stops its motion almost at the beginning of the Aorta, so that the vessels more distant from the heart, are not supplied with blood, sometimes the arteries empty themselves, and the motion of the blood abates, so that at last they become intirely empty Somewhat like this happens in man, in extremity of cold, with loss of pulse, sometimes the want of motion in the arterial blood is joined to their inanition, when there is but few or no globules in the artery · nevertheless we frequently observe a small number of globules, which although distant the one from the other, yet continue their motion.

When the motion of the arterial blood ceaseth, before the strength of the body is exhausted, which is known by the continuation of the motion of the venal blood, there is some hopes that the motion will recover itself without assistance, or by opening a vein This recovery of motion begins by a small number of globules which return into the empty ves-

(*n*) Keill's quantity of blood, p. 91, 92

sel, in a single row their number increaseth by degrees, they dilate the artery which, as it becomes filled with blood, from a pale colour it becomes extremely red, and the blood at last moves therein with much rapidity.

I have often seen (a), as hath also Mr. Lewenhoeck, this recovery of the motion of the artery. We have frequent examples, that arteries filled with blood have lost their motion, which accident hath been easily cured, either by bleeding or without any assistance from art, by the power and effort of the heart only. It often happens in this case, that the grumes of blood formed by globules connected together, are the first that put themselves into motion, whereupon all the blood retakes its course, but we are not always so happy. It is always the case after death, that the arteries empty themselves by degrees, until at last they become absolutely white without the least remains of blood, and become so like the membranes of the Mesentery, that it is very difficult to distinguish the one from the other. After death the motion of the arterial blood is not intirely at an end, until the Mesentery becomes intirely dry, and the globules themselves begin to form dry masses. In animals that have warm blood, it can never be expected that the motions of

(a) Epistle 129 p. 112.

the machine can recover and re-eſtabliſh themſelves, when once the fat becomes fixed.

CHAP IV.

The Motion of the Venal Blood.

I Come now to the motion of the venal blood, in treating whereof I ſhall purſue the ſame order that I obſerved in ſpeaking of the motion of the arterial blood. I will begin with the pulſe, which is generally believed wanting in the veins; yet I have frequently found a pulſe in the large veins of animals that have warm blood. There appeared in 1750, a diſſertation preſented to the royal academy of ſciences at Paris, the author whereof, M Scheighting of Amſterdam, argues for the motion of the brain, againſt people he calls Sophiſts, I was reſolved to examine into this motion, which I did not in the leaſt believe, becauſe of the adheſion of the Dura mater to the Cranium, for this purpoſe, I made a great number of experiments on animals with M. Walſtorf, an able phyſician of Heidelberg, who ſtudied at that time at Gottingen, we eaſily perceived theſe motions, and that they correſponded to thoſe of the lungs, ſo that the brain ſwelled at the time

time of expiration, and subsided at the time of inspiration. I enquired into the cause of this phænomenon, I suspected that it depended on the facility that the blood finds in inspiration, in passing from the right ear into the pulmonary artery, and from the neighbouring veins into this ear. To satisfy myself with respect to the truth of this conjecture, I determined to make some fresh experiments, I laid bare different veins in a living animal, especially the jugulars, the Brachial veins, the Iliacks, and both the Cavæ, I easily perceived they were regularly filled at the time of expiration, becoming then swelled and red by the quantity of blood filling them, and that at the time of inspiration they lengthened themselves, became thin, pale, and empty, and gave no blood on being opened at this time: this I call the venal pulse. I communicated these observations to my friends at France, particularly to M. de Raumur and to M. de Sauvage, from whom M. Lamure must have heard of my experiments. his own words are sufficiently convincing, by the objections (*a*) he sets up against me without naming me (*b*), and by letters which I shall quote. It is concerning this motion of the veins, that I shall now speak,

(*a*) Memoirs of the acad. royal of sciences, 1749 p. 642
(*b*) p. 656.

without knowing what passed at Montpellier, with respect to an essay that I read at the assembly of the society of Gottingen, the 22d of April 1752, and which was printed in the memoirs of the society for this year *(c)*, a little time after M. Walltorf communicated to the public, his experiments as well as mine in an excellent dissertation *(d)*. In this interval of time, M Lamure sent his experiments and thoughts on this motion, to the royal academy of sciences at Paris, in a memoir which was read at one of the assemblies the 12th of August 1752, four months after mine, and which was printed in the memoirs of the year 1749. Some months after the publication of the memoirs of Gottingen, I imagined I ought candidly to report these facts without animosity, in order to prove that I wrote concerning this motion of the veins before M. Lamure *(e)*, and that my expe-

(c) Tom II. p 127.

(d) Dissert qua experimenta circa motum cerebri cerebelli, duræ matris & venerarum in vivis animalibus instituta proposuit Gotting Mens Mart. 1753

(e) This is what the celebrated M de Sauvage hath remarked in a letter dated March 1, 1752, but which was detained in coming, as follows This dog was trepanned, we observed much the motion of the brain, very conformable to that account you have honoured me with, in order to inform me whether the reflux of the blood, during the time of expiration, is the cause of this elevation M. Lamure hath opened above ten dogs, and indeed we have found the same phænomenon as you, and are very much obliged to you for this discovery the original hereof I have by me.

riments

riments have not received any advantage from his. My experiments are much more numerous than those of M. Lamure, and contain many things that I have not found in his memoir, or which are therein contained in a different manner, and yet M. Lamure's memoir contain some facts, which I had not at that time observed. As for example, I was surprised at his good fortune, in having observed the motion of the brain, without detaching the Dura mater from the Cranium, but I have never succeeded in this case (*f*). Secondly, I have observed an alternate motion in the veins of the arm, I have seen another reflux of blood of both the Cavæ, produced by the venal contraction, which I shall speak of in another place. I have observed a motion produced by the contraction of the Diaphragme, also the insensibility of the Dura mater, and other things which are found different in the memoir of M. Lamure, but I have never observed that a ligature, on the jugular veins of a dog, brings on sleep (*g*), or that the sinus's of the brain had any pulse (*h*), and the existence of a space filled with air between the lungs, is disproved by so many experiments, that it seems it never will be confirmed by any pe-

(*f*) Walstorf p. 42, 43, 65.
(*g*) Memoirs of 1749, p. 543, 544.
(*h*) Ibid. p. 547.

netrating wounds of the breast made without wounding the lungs. A weak and vague experiment, on which M Lamure much relieth (*i*).

This ingenious gentleman hath indeed discovered one of the reasons why the jugulars and other veins swell at the time of expiration, which is, because at this time the compression of the breast in general makes the blood flow back from the Cava into the jugulars. I have very lately verified this experiment on a hog (*k*); and, by compressing a long time the Thorax, I have drove back its blood, so as to make the brain swell (*l*). This it was that made me of an opinion, that in expiration, the compression of the breast much contributes to the filling of the veins. not that I would exclude the great facility the blood finds in entering the lungs at the time of inspiration, and which, in this state, takes away the swelling of the veins; nor the other motions which arise from the Diaphragm.

Many facts prove the veins empty themselves at the time of inspiration, by reason of the facility it finds in entering the lungs, and that they fill themselves in expiration, at which time the blood with more difficulty

(*i*) Memoirs of 1749, p 558
(*k*) Ibid p 556 562
(*l*) See the Dissertation of M. Walstorf. p. 39.

enters this Viscus. Hook's experiments, which I have often verified, prove that in lungs that had subsided and become unpassable by inspiration, the blood which had ceased to enter them, and which was not put into motion by the heart, now again enters them, and performs its course.

Injections even succeed better, and pass easier from the pulmonary artery to the vein, when the lungs are inflated. From these observations this consequence may be drawn, which is, that, without the action of inspiration, the blood would with difficulty enter the lungs, and that without expiration, it would cease to move in the veins.

Straining is no more than a retention of the air, and a retarding of expiration. The veins all swell in this interval, and the face becomes swelled and bloated, no doubt, because the blood of the lungs is not expelled, as usual by the action of expiration; and, indeed, without this mechanical compression of the breast, expiration may produce a swelling of the veins, by making a resistance to the passage of the pulmonary artery into the vein, and into the left ventricle. But to these causes of the swelling of the veins, we must, without doubt, add the influence of the contraction of the right auricle; for, besides the swelling of the jugular vein, which is produced by expiration, this vein hath another

other motion much quicker, which resembles a palpitation, and which, if it is carefully observed, is always found at the same time with the first, and which continues after the Thorax is opened, and even after the power of respiration ceaseth. For, it is not only at the distance of some lines, that the right auricle drives back the blood, and receives it again the moment following by alternate contractions and dilatations, but the effect of this motion extends itself even to the liver, under the heart, and above this organ, even to the neck, and in the Mammary veins; and also it appears in a dying animal, and when living in pain, as I have often observed, and which I am actually observing in a cat, now under view.

Lastly, the alternate motion of the Diaphragm occasions the like motion in the Vena Cava, which it drags and tightens as it descends, and in the following expiration it releaseth it, whereupon the vein fills and becomes shortened. All these considerations must be again combined in expounding the motion of the brain and of the veins. Order now requires me to examine the motion of the venal blood, as I have that of the arterial.

For this purpose I have made use of ligatures, after the examples of Harvey and

Walleus *(m)*, who employed this method to prove, contrary to all antiquity, the return of the venal blood to the heart. First I made a ligature on the Cava Inferior near the heart, or on the Superior, or on both at the same time. The effect in both cases is always the same. The blood is collected between the ligatures and the extremities, I mean between the ligature and the limbs, the head, or the Abdomen, but the part of the vein that is intercepted between the auricle and the ligature, remains empty: sometimes these ligatures prevent the motion of the heart, but that does not always happen. As for example, in a frog, I made ligatures on three of the principal veins, in a cat, on the two Cavæ and pulmonary veins, notwithstanding which the heart continued its motions: yet I have observed at other times, in frogs, that the motion of the blood languished extremely on making a ligature on the Cava Inferior *(n)*. However, some error may happen in this observation, for I have seen quite the contrary in the right auricle, which hath drove back the blood into the part that was the nearest to the Vena Cava,

(m) In the Letters de Motu Sanguinis & Chyli, which are found in almost all the Editions of Bartholin's Anatomy, after the year 1641.

(n) See concerning this fact, a dissertation which I have inserted in the first volume of the Memoirs of the Royal Society of Gottingen, p. 273 and the following

and

and propelled it even to the ligature and also into the jugular. This I have seen so often, that it is needless to enumerate the observations on animals on which they were made; and I have observed, since the year 1737, the appearance of a pulse in the jugular vein of a cat, into which the right auricle had discharged some blood even in frogs, this auricle fi'ls very often the Vena Cava with blood, even to the liver, which I shall speak of more at large hereafter.

When a ligature is made on the Vena Cava in the Abdomen, it swells under the ligature; but it does not always become empty between this ligature and the heart, because the blood of the veins and of the liver enters again into that part of the vein, which is between the heart and the ligature. Yet this doth not prevent, in frogs, this portion of the vein from becoming empty. I have tied up the pulmonary veins in the same manner as the two Cavæ, and the effect was the same. The blood collected between the ligature and the lungs, swelled the veins of this Viscus, and that part of the vein that was intercepted between the left ventricle; and the ligature became empty. Sometimes I made a ligature on the Vena Porta, at other times I only tied up the Mesenteric branch. The great Mesenteric vein manifestly swelled (although often very obscurely) between the ligature and the inteſtines; but that part that was between the ligature and the liver was not diminiſhed, and had not leſs blood on being opened, becauſe it is in this intercepted part, that the ſpleinc vein, together with the gaſtric, and ſome others leſs conſiderable, diſcharge their blood.

I afterwards tied up a Meſenteric branch nearer the inteſtines. It ſwelled between the ligature and the inteſtines, but it did not at all diminiſh between the ligature and the liver, becauſe, in this ſpace, a great number of other branches diſcharge their blood, which prevents the perception of any diminution that may happen by any impediment on any ſingle branch. Riolan firſt, and others after him, oppoſed Harvey as to this fact (o) On tying up the jugular vein, I always obſerved the ſpace between the head and the jugular to ſwell, when the other part remained empty, unleſs the force of expiration, and that of the right auricle, had diſturbed the experiment. On tying up the brachial vein of a dog, that part contained between the heart and the ligature became perfectly empty, and ſeemed as fine as a thread, which, on being cut, gave no blood; but the inferior part between the ligature and the paws ſwelled extremely, and gives much blood on opening, but without any pulſation.

(o) Prætermiſſ. the Paris edition, 1652. p. 165

Laſtly,

Lastly, I tied up, in the same manner, the crurale vein of a dog, and that of a great rat; in both the part under the ligature swells, but the part above subsides.

Hence it appears, that always when there are no Anastomosis's supplying blood above the ligature, or when the heart furnisheth none, the blood collects itself between the ligature and the head, the Abdomen or extremities; and that the part between the heart and the ligature becomes entirely empty. This is perfectly consonant to Harvey's discoveries, experiments which, at this time, might be thought unnecessarily repeated, had not Homobon Pisoni, an Italian physician, argued against the circulation; however, truths which are in a manner the foundation of all physic, cannot be too well established. I have never observed, that the veins, when they are tied up, swell so as to become larger than arteries. As they are more flexile, and as the jugular vein, for example, may be dilated by an injection of mercury, so as to form a very large sac; yet, on the other hand, the veins have a greater number of Anastomosis's than the arteries, which serve to convey the blood into the vessels that are free. These anastomosing veins may prodigiously dilate themselves. I have in another place given a description of a vein, which arose from a small vein of one of the ureters, and which,

which, after an obstruction of the Vena Cava, served to carry all the blood from the Iliacs to the Renal, and became as large as the Cava itself.

I have carefully observed the effects of a ligature on the small vessels: for this purpose I have thrice tied up a mesenteric vein in frogs, and, by the assistance of a microscope, I have always found in these experiments, that much blood was collected under the ligature, at which place it lost its motion and fluidity, without making any tumour in the vein; and the blood of the vein passed from the ligature, and returned towards the intestines, and went off by some collateral vein into larger vessels, which brought it to the heart. But when any branch of a vein was entirely filled with fixed blood, in that case the blood of the trunk, without making any effort to dilate this trunk, abandoned the branch that was tied up, and passed into some branch near the ligature. Obstructions of the veins equally assists us, as well as those of the arteries, in accounting for an inflammation, attended with a tumour, redness, and pulsations, which are consequences of the coagulations of the blood, as in a peripneumony.

I now come to speak of what the microscope discovers, with respect to the motion
of

of the venal blood, which I have observed so often in fish and frogs (*p*).

And, first, as to its natural direction: it is as I have before alledged, from the extremities to the heart, so that it passeth from capillary vessels, and of one globule diameter (it seems not consistent to suppose smaller than those) into those of two or three globules diameter, and successively into canals yet larger, and thus cometh to the heart. This I have often carefully, and with much pleasure, observed on the Mesentery of a toad, wherein the Pexus's of the small vessels are more distinct than in a frog.

The motion of the blood in the veins is swift, and (*q*) is not so slow as the major part of physiologists suppose. 'tis also swift in the trunks, and in the ramifications of the veins of an animal in health, and it hath also a swift motion even in the capillary veins. This I have before related, and boldly again declare the same. I might rely on the celebrated M. Musschenbroeck,

(*p*) Malpighy made observations on the Mesentery of a Frog. This celebrated man is the first, who, since the year 1661, that is to say, before Lewenhoeck made observations on the circulation of the blood in the vessels of the lungs. four years afterwards, in 1665, he observed the circulation in the Mesentery of a frog, and established it by very fine observations.

(*q*) See Lewenhoeck, letter 102 and in the continuation of his Arcan. Natur. p. 131.

who faith, that the motion of the arterial blood is very swift at the place where these vessels degenerate into veins (r). But 'tis best to use no other proofs than those of experiments; in the greater part of those which I have made with respect to the veins, I have observed that the velocity of their blood was not so great as that of the blood of the correspondent arteries, but about three times slower, for the veins have generally their light or cavities about three times larger than the arteries. Nevertheless, it often happens, that no difference is at all perceived between the velocity of the arterial blood and that of the venal blood in the correspondent vessels. I have even sometimes found a greater velocity in the vein, and 'tis observed often, that the veins preserve their motion after the arteries have lost theirs. In general, there is no occasion of any calculation to prove that the velocity of the blood in both the Cavæ. is to the velocity of the blood of the Aorta, in an inverse proportion to the size of these vessels, and the sizes and magnitudes of both the Cavæ are not quite three times larger than the Aorta, the proportion of 3578 to 1000, established by Dr Clifton Wintringham much exceeds the truth, because it makes the ratio of the diameter of the Superior Cava as 1865 to 1000, al-

(r) Essais Physique, p 392.

though in man the Aorta is rather larger than the Cava Superior. Sometimes the small vessels and the capillary veins seem to bring back the blood with less velocity (s) than the trunks, and the velocities seem to be almost in a direct proportion to their magnitudes: and I have sometimes found, that when two capillary vessels re-united, so as to form but one trunk, that the velocity increased in this re-united branch. As in general, if the velocity of the blood in the Aorta becomes less in the capillary arteries, it must follow that the velocity the blood hath in the capillary veins must increase in the large ones (t): I have, nevertheless, sometimes observed, that this velocity was greater in the capillary veins than in the trunks. This diminution of velocity in the small vessels, make the globules seem separated and at a greater distance the one from the other, and this distance is pretty considerable: but, in the great vessels, the globules seem to form a continued mass, and this separation of the globules produceth no diminution of their velocities. These vessels must certainly contain some other fluid that is invisible, which forms the chain of connection between each red globule, without

(s) Malpighi, in his work before cited, p. 92.
(t) Butler of Blood-letting, p. 11. Robinson Animal. Oeconom. prop. 10.

which it would be impossible to conceive how the force of the heart could propel the globules in a continual succession, and, moreover, because the veins are destitute of any contraction, and cannot assist the motion of these globules

The venal blood, moving with less velocity, is more subject to lose its motion than the arterial, and more easily becomes retrograde, which I shall hereafter more fully relate; yet we often observe it to preserve its motion longer than the blood of the arteries, as I have before observed.

These two motions differ, for the motion of the venal blood does not (as far at least as I have been able to observe) undergo any accelaration either in the small or large vessels (*u*), but moves every where with an equal velocity, and it flows with the same equality of motion, when a vein is opened (*x*). I have nothing to do in this place with the respiratory pulse, of which I have already spoken, nor with that species of pulse which the retrocession of the blood of the auricle produceth in the Vena Cava, nor with that revived velocity which the venal blood acquires sometimes after it had been entirely at rest, or at least after an accidental decrease of velocity.

(*u*) G. Adams, before cited, p 45
(*x*) J. A. Borelli de Motu Animalium, lib. 2. prop 31.

It is observable in the veins, and even more distinctly than in the arteries, that the globules that move in the middle of the vessels in the axis, have a somewhat greater velocity than those which move nearer the parieties (y). I have not found that any angles of the vessels diminished the velocity of the circulation; but, on the contrary, I have observed, in places where the vessels communicate, that the blood passed from the one to the other, under very acute angles, with as much rapidity as it did before.

The retrocession of the blood-globules against the parieties, at the division of two veins, is made without any effort or resilition; and, in this place, they pass into the branch without changing their form, and continue their natural course: and these oscillatory fuctions of two columns, proceeding one against another, neither change their direction of a right line, nor the form of the globules.

No rotating or winding motion is observed in the veins; for all the venal blood is moved in right lines (z), parallel the one to the other. And, although the different appearances of the globules, which, in the capillary vessels, seem sometimes transparent,

(y) Malpighi Posthum p 92
(z) Malpighi, the work before cited, p 92.

and

and sometimes opake, and seem to shew a rotating motion, yet these different appearances depend much more on the flexions of these small vessels, than on any real change in the globules.

As Anastomosis's are by far more frequently observed in the large veins than in the arteries, and, as there is found a large network of veins in the Mesentery of frogs, it affords an opportunity of confirming what I have said concerning the ramifications of the vessels: it is certain, the blood moves in them sometimes in its natural direction, and sometimes in a contrary direction (*a*). When two venal trunks communicate together by any neighbouring branch, sometimes one of the trunks, and sometimes the other furnisheth this communicating vessel with blood; and this happens even in a healthy state I speak not here of any preternatural oscillations; and the following phænomenon is worth taking notice of, which is, That if a small vein hath its insertion in a venal trunk much larger, the force of the current of this large vessel entirely stops the motion of the blood of the small vein, although it is of some globules diameter, and hinders it from conveying its blood into the great trunk. This teacheth us, why nature hath ordered, that the veins of one globule dia-

(*a*) De Heide Observ. 85.

meter are never inserted into trunks much larger than themselves, and, why very small branches re-unite, and form little trunks, which, afterwards re-uniting and forming a larger trunk, make a successive gradation, thereby giving to the blood of the larger branches a force sufficient to enter the trunks, notwithstanding the resisting force of their currents. This shews the necessity of the thoracic duct, and strengthens the opinion I have, that a small lymphatic vein does not convey its blood into the Vena Cava; the lumbar vein, or the Azygos, as Pecquet, in his last experiments (*b*), Kulmus, and some others, have supposed.

The disorders which the circulation of the venal blood undergoes are, as in the arteries, its perturbation, oscillation, retrogradation, its want of motion, and, sometimes, manition, although this last is much less frequent than in the arteries

The perturbation of motion in the venal blood consists (as in the arteries) in this; its motion diminisheth, and afterwards it recovers its velocity, sometimes it stops entirely, and afterwards it recovers its motion with an increased velocity. Perhaps these irregularities and uncertainties in the velocity of the venal blood, made M. Quesnay *(c)* declare

(*b*) Nouvelle Insertion du Canal Thorachique.
(*c*) Oeconomie Animal, first edition, p 233

That

That nothing certain could be established on this article.

The oscillation in the veins is a beautiful phænomenon, as well by reason of the magnitude of the venal network and Plexus's, but because the venal blood, in all my experiments, appeared to be very subject to a retrograde motion, which necessarily produceth an oscillation that remains as long as sufficient strength is preserved to keep up the motion in the other vessels.

The venal blood alternately moveth backward and forward in the same trunk, and sometimes moves back to the intestines, before it returns to the heart. This is very frequently observed in fish and frogs, when these animals begin to grow languid. The blood seems to meet with some obstacle and resistance in the trunk, whereby it is forced back, and, as it goes back from the trunk, it is stopped by the force of the blood of the branch, but before it changeth its direction, some opposition is observed: for, the columns of blood, which follow opposite currents, run against and mutually repel each other. At other times, I have observed a trunk of the Mesentery to convey the blood even to the middle of the Mesentery, from whence it returned to the intestines by another trunk, whose blood had the same direction as that of the arteries.

On the other hand, I have found, in places where two transverse branches were inserted into the same trunk, that the blood balanced itself in the manner following: sometimes, for a moment, it had a motion of retrogradation from the trunk into one or other of the branches, and presently following its natural motion, it moved from two branches into the trunk, at other times, being repelled from the branch on the right side, it went retrograde through the trunk into the left branch, from whence it returned through the trunk into the branch on the right side; and this I have observed for above thirty minutes.

But the veins which communicate with each other, and in which the blood is seen to move in all possible directions, afford a more beautiful observation. The blood of a vein near the heart, and on the right side, passeth by a middle trunk into a trunk placed more to the left side, and the resistance which it there finds, produceth an oscillation, after this oscillation, it descends by the left trunk towards the intestines, or else it takes again its former course by the middle trunk: sometimes, in going out of this vessel, it takes its natural course by moving towards the heart, at other times, it becomes retrograde under the insertion of the vessel of communication. Sometimes the motion beginning

ginning by a trunk on the right side near the intestines, the blood passeth first by an Anastomosis into a trunk on the left side, from whence it takes its course, sometimes to the heart, and sometimes downwards towards the intestines (d), or else it continues its motion in its trunk towards the heart, according to the common course of circulation: also, in the same venal trunk, 'tis observed, that one part of the blood carried thereto from a ramification, moves towards the heart, and another part at the same time towards the intestines What I have said with respect to the trunk of the right side, soon after happens in the left trunk: sometimes the blood returns thereto, and sometimes it passeth by the middle canal, from whence it is either brought to the heart, or repelled towards the intestines. The difference of the angles, which the middle branch makes with the two trunks, creates no difference in the velocity of the blood in its passing from these two vessels; and it passeth from the left trunk under an acute angle, with as great a velocity as it had at it's first passing from the trunk on the right side under an obtuse angle. I have distinctly observed this kind of conflict taking place between the different columns, which are carried away by their motion; so that this direct and indirect mo-

(d) De Heide hath perceived somewhat like this

tion of the blood produceth a sort of confusion in the vessels (*e*). And I have very often found, as I have said elsewhere, that of all the vessels, there are none in which the motion is longer continued than in the branches of communication.

Moreover, I have seen in one and the same venal trunk, and three of its branches, the following different motions. In the trunk there was an oscillation: one moment the blood moved retrograde, the next moment, as it moved from the part the nearest to the intestines, it was carried in its natural direction towards the heart, or at least into some branch conveying the blood that way. The superior branch contained but few globules, but they had a very remarkable oscillatory motion, so that they were alternately carried towards the intestines, and the next moment towards the heart. With respect to the middle branch, the blood of the trunk sometimes entered it, and, at other times, it was repelled from thence very strongly. Lastly, after the blood had descended with a great velocity into the inferior trunk, it afterwards relinquished the same, and ascended against its own weight. All this was observed after I had divided two of the principal trunks of the Aorta.

(*e*) This is the motion that so much surprized Lewenhoeck, Contin. Arcan. Natur. p. 116.

Sometimes an oscillation ariseth in the following manner. The blood ceaseth entirely its motion, and recovers it again in a retrograde direction, and it passeth again into some other branch, by which it returns to the heart (*f*). The direct and natural motion sometimes succeeds an oscillation, and at other times a retrogradation is followed by a total cessation of motion, which generally happens, as I shall relate elsewhere, when the heart is taken away. It seems that it is to this oscillatory motion, that the celebrated M. Whytt attributes the motion of the blood in the small vessels (*g*), but this opinion will be destroyed, if we consider that this motion never takes place in an animal in health, and that it cannot be reckoned among the natural causes of the motion of the blood, but is preternatural, and a disease.

Nothing is more frequent than the retrograde motion of the venal blood, and often when a frog is observed with a microscope, and the arteries are found to keep up very regularly their pulsations, yet the venal blood begins to turn back, and return to the intestines, they having no valves to oppose it, I am apt to think that a wound is often the cause of this retrogradation, because the re-

(*f*) Malpighi in the same place, p. 92.
(*g*) On Vital Motion, p. 96.

flux of the blood is very common when any venous veffel happens to break; I own it fometimes takes place, although no veffel is open, fometimes a coalition of the blood occafions it (*h*): and this is evident, becaufe the natural motion again takes place after the diffolution of the coagulum that was formed by the red globules. At other times I have feen the blood repelled by the grumous blood of a vein that was divided: I have alfo feen the blood return from a large trunk into a fmall branch of fome globules diameter. This is what a friend of the celebrated M. Baker took for the fecretion of fome extreme fine humour (*i*).

The ofcillation, and the motion of retrogradation, are almoft always followed by a ceffation of motion, but this is not of any continuance, provided the vital ftrength is not impaired: and, in this cafe the blood, which was before at reft, is obferved to put itfelf again into motion, in order to purfue its natural courfe. In animals that have warm blood, the motion of the blood ceafeth much fooner, and the veins of the Abdomen, that is opened in a living animal, become varicous and fwelled by the collection of the blood that had loft its motion, as the

(*h*) As in the example mentioned by Lewenhoeck, Experim & Contemp p 208
(*i*) See this author's work, before cited, p 136

great Boerhaave demonstrated to his auditors. This cessation of motion begins in the small vessels, in fish it begins in those that are the nearest the tail, in frogs, in the network and ramifications of veins of one globule diameter, although the blood in the great trunks at the same time continueth its motion (*). Sometimes the motion ceaseth in some branches, and continues in others; and indeed it hath happened, that small veins, of one or two globules diameter, preserve their motion, after it hath entirely ceased, not only in the trunks of the veins, but also in the larger arteries. I have observed in a Toad, that the small vessels preserved their motion, although I had taken away the heart, but this seldom happens. When the blood is at rest, the veins are often very full, and this blood, by reason of its Striæ, resembles oil, and the day after death, I have found the veins full of blood, that was dry and immoveable: yet, sometimes the veins appear empty at the beginning of the experiment, by reason of the animal's fasting, or of some other cause. In other subjects, they are only empty in some particular part, and in others, they contain blood in their whole extent, but in a small quantity and of a yellow colour. Lastly, after apparent death, the veins are generally

(*) See De Heide Exper. 8.

either

either empty, or at most but one half full, especially if the animal had lost a little blood: also, 'tis not seldom we find in animals that have warm blood, and even in man, veins either empty or filled with Bullæ of air, either in the brain or other parts. Almost all authors that have treated on this subject, make the veins full of blood after death; which is true with respect to the Vena Cava, and the other large vessels, into which the blood is forced by cold or other causes (of which I shall speak in the sixth chapter); and, by this means, there is a congestion of blood at the entrance into the lungs, but this is not constant in the smaller veins.

CHAP. V.

The Effects of Bleeding in the Course and Direction of the Blood.

I Employed myself in anatomy at Paris, when M. Silva, who was in considerable repute among the practitioners there, published his treatise on bleeding; a work that met with a multitude of opponents. His system was founded on this principle of Bellini, who said, That when a vein is opened, the blood of that vein, as also that of the neighbouring veins, and also that of the artery that furnisheth them with blood, acquires a new degree of velocity, and projects itself towards the orifice. By this means a great derivation of the humours is made on the part where the vein is opened, and the other veins, which have no communication therewith, undergo by this means a considerable revulsion.

Many authors (*a*) opposed this doctrine, but especially M. Quesnay (*b*); and with him a person of a superior genius, the celebrated M. Senac, who, in his letters published under the fictitious name of Julian Morisson (*c*), and afterwards in his medical essays on the anatomy of M. Heister, and, lastly, in his treatise on the heart, hath, with much honour, opposed the Bellinian doctrine. As to the practising physicians, some have followed the ancient doctrine, and some are friends to the new one. Since this I have been desirous of satisfying myself by

(*a*) M. Chevalier Observations Critiques sur le Traité des Saignees, 12. 1730. M. Roger Butler Essay on Blood-letting, 8. London 1734. Brown Langrish modern Theory and Practice of Physick, 8. London 1738. M. Martin de la Phlebotomie & de l'Arteriotomie, 12. Paris 1741. M. Roland Jackson de Vera Phlebotomiæ Theoria, 8. London 1747. Giles Watts of Revulsion and Derivation, 8. London 1754.

(*b*) Observations sur la Saignee, 12. Paris 1730.

(*c*) Lettres sur le Choix des Saignees, 12. Paris 1730.

experiments, what real changes bleeding could produce with respect to the course of the blood; nothing seemed more proper to decide this controversy, than to bleed a living animal, that we may be able to distinguish the blood through the membranes of the veins, and observe the changes it at this time undergoes. For this reason, I was determined to take the method which M. de Heide had began, and to add new experiments to those he hath left us, and which have their use. I have made use of a great number of animals in these experiments; some whereof were made with M. Remus, and the major part of them I made in the summer-time of the year 1754. Bleeding, by opening the veins, is not attended with much difficulty in a man of a little experience; for the mesenteric veins of frogs, and of toads especially, are very visible, and are easily opened with a lancet: but bleeding by opening of the arteries, which are smaller, not so high coloured, and harder, is not quite so easily performed; yet I have opened a great many, and I do not at all regret the time I have employed in making these experiments.

The first thing I was to examine was, whether the velocity of the blood increased in the vein that is opened, and in its adjacent ones. This supposition being the foundation of all the Bellinian theory (*d*), if it is not true, the whole system is destroyed. The celebrated author, under the name of Julian Morisson (*e*), absolutely denies that the blood moves with a greater velocity from the vein that is opened, than from those that are intire, or that bleeding produceth any acceleration in the motion of the venal blood. The late M Hamberger maintains in a manner the same sentiments; for he reckons the augmentation of the velocity, produced by bleeding only, as 200 to 201 (*f*). As for my part, I have very often observed, and as often as I desired, the result having been always the same I say I have observed, that whatever the direction of the blood was, in the vein that I opened, whether it moved in its natural course to the heart, or whether by any retrograde motion it was carried towards the intestines, or whether it was upon the poise or at rest, or, lastly, whether the heart was taken away, or the Aorta's tied up or divided In all these cases, the blood issued from the vein that was opened with a velocity much greater than that which

(*d* Proposit 1
e, See the fifth letter, also a thesis read at Paris, in 1734, on this subject, when Baron was president, and Les Essais de Physique, edit of 1735. p 522 524
(*f*) Dissertatio de Ven Sect n 43

it

it had in the intire vein (g), and even with a greater than it hath in the arteries. At first it issues from the vein in winding motions, as if it was propelled by the weight of a large column of water, sufficient to force and strain the tube, and its velocity, which is the greater at the wound, diminisheth, in proportion as the blood extravasates into the Laminæ of the Mesentery, and the globules, which were at first collected together, so as to form but a very small passage, by degrees separate themselves, and the channel of the current becomes considerably larger. Two opposite currents, both swift in motion, hasten to the orifice of the vein, yet there comes more blood, and with a greater velocity from the heart, and the column that comes from thence, repelling that which comes from the extremities, furnisheth almost all the blood which is lost by bleeding.

Afterwards I observed that the opening of a vein produceth a very swift motion of the venal blood, even after it hath been a long time at rest (h), and the heart taken away, and that this velocity takes place not only in the vein that is opened, and the branches communicating therewith, but also

(g) These experiments are conformable to those of De Heide. See his work, p. 2. 4.

(h) See De Heide, p. 4. 8. and Hale's Hæmastatics, p. 165.

in the adjacent trunks that communicate with it, and even in the small capillary veins. This experiment I always make with success, unless the vein that is opened hath lost all its blood, or is become dry: it also succeeds, as I have before declared, after the heart is taken away; and after a ligature is made on the two great trunks of the Aorta, from which the whole body of this animal receives its blood. Lastly, bleeding seems to have so great a power to vary the course of the blood, that it produceth a motion contrary to the common laws of circulation (1) it makes the blood move retrograde from the heart towards the incision, and it accelerates the motion of that which was coming from the intestines; this produceth in the orifice an influx of blood from two opposite columns. 'Tis entertaining to observe this opposition, arising between these two columns; and this is sometimes the more distinct, as they are of different colours: for the current from the heart is of a much deeper red than that which comes from the intestines, which is more pale.

This rapid motion considerably, and almost entirely emptieth the adjacent veins, as the blood which returneth from the heart, hath a greater velocity than that which

(1) De Heide, p 5 8.

cometh from the inteſtines, its motion is continued longer; and this difference of velocity and duration is nearly in the ſame proportion: ſometimes the current from the heart only ſupplieth the blood.

The adjacent veins empty themſelves towards the inciſion, not only by a direct, but alſo by a retrograde motion (*k*). And, if their blood ceaſeth its motion, bleeding reſtores it; and, at the ſame time, gives a fluidity to the congeſtion of globules, which this want of motion had cauſed to degenerate into a kind of oily maſs.

After having made two orifices in one vein, between which the blood was at reſt, and at neither of which orifices the blood diſcharged itſelf, I obſerved at laſt it determined itſelf towards the inferior orifice, by which it went out.

There happens but little alteration, either with reſpect to the velocity, or with reſpect to the evacuation in the veins of the Meſenſentery that are the moſt diſtant from thoſe which are opened, as hath been juſtly obſerved by the author of thoſe letters under the name of Moriſſon (*l*). The congeſtions of the re-united globules recover their motion by bleeding, and the grumes which ſometimes diſcharge themſelves at the orifice

(*k*) De Heide, p 4
(*l*) Lettre huit Eſſais de Phyſique, p. 526. 529.

like red clouds, contribute to re-eſtabliſh a free circulation. Laſtly, and what is not commonly obſerved after ſeven times bleeding, I have ſeen the motion of the venal blood to continue for two hours even in the ſmall capillary veſſels. By all this it appears, how neceſſary bleeding is to re-eſtabliſh any ſuſpended circulation in perſons drowned, and in ſoporiferous diſtempers.

Alſo it appears, that bleeding brings the blood from the adjacent part into that where this operation is performed, and that therefore there is nothing in the doctrine of derivation that is contradictory to experiments, provided its effect is not hindered by the valves. Thus bleeding in the jugular emptieth the heart, the right auricle, and the lungs, becauſe there are no valves oppoſing this. I am convinced of by other experiments on a dog, in which I ſaw diſtinctly, that the blood found no obſtacle from the right auricle into the external jugular. It is yet more certain, and more generally known, that bleeding in this vein eaſeth the brain.

We ſee alſo that the coagulums produced, as great men have obſerved, by fear, cold, fevers, or other cauſes, may be diſſolved and removed by bleeding, and that it gives a fluidity to the blood that was at reſt.

It

It is not only in any particular part, but even in all the animal body, that the coagulated and viscid blood may be resolved by this increase of velocity, which bleeding produceth, as any one may find by experiments on frogs.

Another theorem may be drawn from these facts, which is, that, as all the veins of the body are connected to one another, the nearest to those which are opened, empty themselves the most, and those which are more distant, discharge themselves into the former, their blood acquires a velocity somewhat greater: but these effects always diminish in proportion to the distance from the vein that is opened, and at length absolutely cease (*m*). For, as every hæmorrhage stops soon enough without assistance, and in artificial bleedings the blood very soon stops, even without any bandage, therefore it never happens that all the veins entirely empty themselves; and those which are distant from the orifice, empty themselves but very little, as I have related in giving the result of the experiment. Although derivation, and even a small revulsion in the veins, are proved by these facts, yet they are not sufficient to prove

(*m*) A man of a great genius, M G C Oeder profession at Copenhagen, hath cleared up this matter in his Inaugural Thesis, published at Gottingen, ann 1749.

that these effects are produced in the utmost extremities of the body.

But the second, and most important part of the question is, to know whether bleeding accelerates, also the motion of the arterial blood as laid down in the Bellinian doctrine (*n*). What proves in effect the importance of this part of the question is, that 'tis not on the derivation, or the revulsion of the veins, that we depend in practice, but on that which ought to be made by the arteries corresponding with the vein that is opened. For inflammatory distempers, as phrensies and the pleurisy, are considered as diseases of the arteries; and, lastly, the great Boerhaave, and with him almost all practitioners, expect by opening a vein, to determine that way the course of the blood, which swells the inflamed part, and to remove obstructions from the extremities of the arteries, and return a fluidity to the blood, it is very difficult to decide this question by experiments; their result hath not been always the same, and that which I have made on myself, did not answer my expectation. For in a continual fever, many of which, and very troublesome ones, I laboured under at Gottingen, I was blooded. before the

---

(*n*) See Bellini, propos 1 and H Schulze, in a dissertation, intitled, Prejudic circa Ven Sect Opinion &c.

operation, my pulse had 122 pulsations in a minute, it retained the same velocity during the operation, and after it was finished. As to making experiments on living animals, there is another difficulty attends it, which is, that the motion of the arteries decreaseth more slowly than that of the veins, and we must wait many hours before this diminution becomes sensible, and, unless you wait for this diminution of motion, the motion of the arterial blood, which is of itself swift, becomes not accelerated by bleeding, and, if you defer the operation, until the motion of the arterial blood is slackened, often, in this interval, the veins become dry and empty, and are no more proper for the experiment.

I intend honestly to report the results of sixty-two experiments. In thirty-six, I have not considered the arterial blood; or, at least, its velocity was too great to be augmented by bleeding. In twenty-six others, I carefully observed the change produced in them by this operation. In five bleedings I could not find any alteration was produced thereby, with respect to the motion of the blood in the corresponding artery; and with respect to the adjacent arteries, there was only one of them in which, either by the effect of bleeding or of some other cause, the blood of the artery moved a little slower after the operation.

In

In twenty-one other cases, bleeding increased the motion in the arteries, either if it was only diminished or totally suspended: sometimes it began again its motion by balancing itself, at other times it successively recovered its natural motion an hour after it had been at rest, both the arterial and venal blood moved pretty swiftly, and this motion was increased by bleeding even in the arteries themselves.

Eight of these experiments were made on animals which had but little or no blood in the adjacent arteries, and when the blood began to run out of the orifice of the vein, a greater quantity of blood entered the artery, and its velocity increasing with the quantity, it presently became full, and this happened after I had taken away the heart.

I have observed that the blood which was at rest in an Aneurisme, produced by Arteriotomy, and also that the blood in the adjacent artery was put into motion by bleeding, and flowed, though in a small stream, through the Aneurisme and the trunk, it afterwards stopped its motion, and some globules were observed to have a retrograde motion in the artery. A second bleeding in the correspondent vein procured again a direct motion in the artery, and the trunk from which it took its rise. When a vein is opened after death, or after the

heart

heart is taken away, it produceth some motion in the artery.

By what I have related, it appears that the cases wherein bleeding hath increased the motion of the artery, are more numerous than those wherein it hath not; therefore no regard is to be had to the objection I am now endeavouring to prevent. These increased motions, you may say, have not their sole cause from bleeding; but they have too frequently happened after it, to attribute them to any other accidental cause. Why, in effect, should this happen the very moment of bleeding? Therefore we may conclude with respect to the second question, without any doubt, that after bleeding, the motion of the blood is accelerated in the correspondent arteries bordering on the vein that is opened. And my experiments confirm the Bellinian doctrine on derivation, which prove, that when a vein is opened, the blood supplies more abundantly the arteries of the part where the vein hath been opened: the objection which may be made with respect to the valves, in the prior experiments on the veins, have no force against these last.

What fully establisheth the revulsion of the artery, is, that the blood collecting in the place where the vein is opened, and the quantity of the whole mass not increasing at this time, the arteries bordering on those which

which are discharged by the orifice, empty their blood into these last, finding therein the least resistance, and this diminution of resistance taking place in the contiguous vessels, the effect must be extended to arteries at some distance; yet it doth not follow, that it should extend to those at a much greater distance, because the small Anastomosis's between two, are not sufficient to create a very swift motion of the blood of one artery to another that is very distant; so it cannot be expected that the blood of the brain can throw itself on the crural artery through the small Anastomosis's of the spinal marrow, or of the vessels of the bason (*o*).

And if, moreover, we add to this, that a man becomes weak by losing blood, and that the force of the heart being diminished, whereby the resistance which is made by the arteries in the parts opposite to that wherein bleeding is performed, is found proportionably greater than in a man in health It is a just doctrine to determine a greater quantity of blood to the parts whose vein is opened, rather than to the brain or other parts, wherein nothing hath diminished the resistance of the vessels. We see then, that derivation and

---

(*o*) It will appear in the Fasciculi Iconum 4 plate 4, and 7 That the arteries of the Coccyx and Sacrum are united with the arteries of the spinal marrow by frequent Anastomosis s

revulfion are proved by thefe experiments; for there arifeth a true revulfion from the head, always when lefs blood is carried thither from the heart, and thereby the veffels of the brain are confequently lefs fwelled.

I confefs that all this is true only during the time of bleeding; but when the orifice is clofed, all, as I fhall declare prefently (*p*), enter again into their prior ftate and uniformity (*q*): but the motion of the blood almoft always lofeth fomewhat of its force and velocity, which is another great intention, and even what commonly phyficians aim at, when they direct bleeding in fevers. For, the grand point is, to reduce the exceffive force of the heart, which hardens the coagulum, and fills the veffels already too much dilated, and occafions dangerous extravafations from the obftructed veffels into the cellular membrane, and alfo increafeth, by a great heat, a tendency in the blood to a volatile putrefcency. It remains for me now to confider the other phænomena which happen when a vein is opened.

I made two incifions in the fame vein; the fuperior, which was the neareft the heart, retarded the flowing of the blood by

(*p*) See De Heide, p 8
(*q*) Bellini fuppofeth, propof 11. That the velocity is greater after bleeding than before, but this is not confonant to experiments.

the inferior incision, but it did not suppress it. You find by this experiment, what may be expected by bleeding, in order to stop a hæmorrhage. It acts chiefly by weakening the action of the heart, whose force we endeavour to diminish, until the hæmorrhage stops naturally, or until remedies may be applied for that purpose.

The stream of blood issuing from the vein, by degrees slackens, and the globules, which with force separated themselves in different directions, collect themselves round the wound, so that it becomes surrounded with a large spot, the colour whereof is always the less red in the places the more distant from the orifice of the vein, and more red in those that are nearer thereto. We observe also in the wound the grume, whereof I have spoken in the second chapter. This grume is formed by the re-union of the red globules, which I have observed in a vein that I opened by the side of the Mesentery that was the nearest to the glass, and which intersects the middle of a tubercle, that is white and membranous, fixed to the vein.

After the orifice of the vein is closed, the blood re-assumes its former motion, sometimes it moves in a direction from the heart, when the grume is taken away by friction,
the

the wound opens again, and the hæmorrhage returns (r). Sometimes the current re-establisheth itself in the vein, so as to fill the vessel; at other times it begins by two or three small distinct torrents, carried through the white cloud. If one half of the vein is divided by incision, this orifice remains open; and yet, what is very surprising, the circulation is continued above this orifice, by the small portion of the canal which is preserved.

If the vein is entirely tore, sometimes no blood issues from it, but, in this case, the vein either closeth itself at its extremity, like a round tuberosity full of viscid blood, or else it forms a kind of cone closed at the Apex, in which the blood becomes fixed. I have at this time observed the coagulated blood to repel that which came from the heart, and which went to the extremity of the vein and made an oscillation with that blood, but, sometimes when it is a considerable vein which hath been thus divided, it gives blood abundantly. When a vein is intirely cut, sometimes it gives blood from the seat of the heart, at other times it gives none, espe-

(r) See De Heide, p 3 By this we see how necessary rest is in wounds of the vessels, and what care ought to be taken not to cleanse them too roughly, for fear of destroying that favourable grume that closeth the mouth of the artery

cially if the animal is a little feeble, it forms at its extremities a fack full of blood, which begins to balance itself by moving backwards and forwards with that which moves retrograde from the heart.

The opening of an artery produceth nearly the fame phænomena with thofe of a vein, but the motion of the arterial blood being much more fwift than that of the venal, it iffues from the wound with a velocity much greater: it is furprifing; and this velocity is greater than it was before the incifion.

The opening of an artery equally accelerates the motion of the blood, as well in the artery that is opened, as in the correfpondent ones; and this acceleration extends to a confiderable diftance. From the incifion, we obferve to iffue not only the blood which comes from the feat of the heart, but alfo a column, which, by a retrograde (s) motion, returns from the inteftines, and which makes itfelf a paffage, notwithftanding the refiftance it meets with from the column which comes from the heart.

When either the heart or the Aorta is cut off, generally the blood of the mefenteric artery moves retrograde; this artery emptieth itfelf, and a perfect reft enfues: yet I have obferved, in opening this mefenteric artery, that the fmall number of red globules, which

(s) See De Heide, p 3 6

were diſtributed in all its extent, and which filled but a ſmall part of it, continued to flow.

When the blood ceaſeth to flow from the wound, for this happens eſpecially if the animal is weak, and a ſecond inciſion is made in the artery higher than the firſt, it revives the motion of the blood, and eſtabliſheth it, as well between the two inciſions as under the firſt (*t*).

After the current of blood flows from the wound in the artery, the motion of the blood by degrees abates, and is diſcompoſed; and we obſerve globules, either ſlowly to move one by one, or a new wave coming intire from the heart: but the column which comes from the inteſtines the firſt, becomes weak, and, after ſome conteſt, the force of the column from the ſeat of the heart prevailing, at laſt repels the other, and compelling it to retake its courſe under the wound, it puts again the motion of the blood into its natural ſtate.

The wound of an artery cloſeth itſelf in the ſame manner as that of a vein: there becomes formed under the inciſion a kind of ſmall ſpot, like a cloud, which at firſt is red, afterwards it changeth, and becomes pale about its edges. In the middle a grume is formed by the re-union of ſome globules, the motion of the blood by degrees abates,

(*t*) De Heide hath obſerved ſomething like this, p. 7.

even in the artery, until this fluid, having passed beyond the grume, takes up again its former course

It is very certain, that it is a coagulated fluid which closeth the wound of the artery. I have observed red globules to force a passage through this cloud, and flow out of the wound into the Laminæ of the Mesentery, and the hæmorrhage returned by rubbing the artery, and taking away the gluten which closeth the wound When the incision is large, it preserves its diameter without diminution, and it doth not become smaller by any contraction: after the wound is healed, the blood takes again its natural motion (u), or rather a motion somewhat more flow, often all the blood of the arteries flows out of the incision, and they remain entirely empty (x)

It is not uncommon to find an artery that hath been opened, more dilated in the place of the Cicatrix, and an Aneurisme formed there. I cut an Aneurisme of this kind, but nothing flowed from it; and I observed a membrane, surrounding it circularly with a small opening, obstructed by a small grume of blood. I saw this blind sack to fill by degrees with blood, and which came from a column from the heart, as being the strongest,

. See De Heide, p 8 (x) Ibid. p 3 6.

as soon as it was filled, the blood passed beyond and entered an adjacent branch.

There is also another way whereby wounds of the arteries close themselves, and that is by the contraction of their membrane, not that it is muscular, for nothing of this appears in the arteries of frogs, but by a natural contraction which brings the fibres towards the Axis, and draws them from the contact of the rest of the membrane, and which takes place even in the arteries of a dead subject.

An artery that is tore and not cut, contracts itself and forms a round tumour, from which I have sometimes observed there did not issue one drop of blood, although it was supplied with it from a neighbouring branch; at other times it gave blood. This makes me believe, that the umbilical arteries of a fœtus that is strong, would bleed if they were cut, unless a ligature is used, and that those of a fœtus that was weak would not. Therefore the experiments of the late M. Schuize, who supposed that without any danger the binding and tying up the chord might be omitted, and those of his adversaries who have seen bad consequences by this neglect, may be equally true. I have observed on the fœtus of a cat that had been four weeks pregnant, which fœtus I took from the cat by the cesarean operation, that the umbilical arteries always beat when

when the heart of this little animal contracted itself (y).

When the artery and the vein are opened at the same time, the blood flows equally from both, but there is no alteration in its velocity. The blood of the mesenterick artery of a sheep spurted six feet high, I opened another artery, at which time the spring of neither exceeded one foot.

Moreover I have observed, that on opening the great vessels of dogs or sheep, the first spring of the blood only extends itself to a certain height, which diminisheth considerably after the first, and it is only with respect to this first spring of the blood, on which the calculations are founded, whereby we endeavour to consider the motion of the heart.

CHAP. VI.

Of the Causes of the Motion of the Blood.

THERE is yet remaining the most difficult part of the work, which is, to discover the causes producing all these different motions which I have hitherto described.

(y) M Smelhe, an excellent midwife, hath observed in infants where the Funis hath not been sufficiently bound, that a very considerable quantity of blood was lost. In his cases and observations,

The

The heart is generally allowed to be the firſt; to which is added the contraction of the arteries, the compreſſion of the muſcles, the action of the nerves; and ſome authors beſides add thereto the ſuction of the capillary veſſels. Beſides the effects of theſe different powers, I will enquire into the effects of weight, of cold and heat, of the internal air, and laſtly into the effects of that unknown power, for which I ſhall preſerve the name of attraction, until new experiments ſhall better diſcover to us its nature, for all theſe cauſes act independent of the heart, and produce conſiderable motions in the blood. The motion of the heart is certainly the principal agent of the motion of the blood, in animals that have cold blood: this fluid, I confeſs, preſerves its motion for 40 minutes after the heart is taken away, and even longer, by the power of the cauſe I have laſt mentioned; but the order and conſtancy of theſe motions, even in animals of this kind, ceaſe immediately by deſtroying the heart, whoſe want of motion produceth the ſame effect in all the other parts of the animal body, and whoſe motion re eſtabliſheth all the others; all the humours return unto and go from the heart. In animals that have warm blood, its motion hardly ſubſiſts one minute after the heart is deſtroyed. A motion of this conſequence, deſerves a very careful examination, even in

the

the different states of the blood's motion, I will, in this inquiry, only consult experiments (*a*). and I shall not mention the opinions of different authors, who have treated on this subject, which would extend this work to an excessive length.

It may be said, that the motion of the heart begins at one of the Venæ Cavæ for, when we tie up or cut these veins, the motion of the right auricle, and that of the right ventricle, soon abates, and presently intirely ceaseth, these veins are by nature the first agent of the heart's motion.

There is a considerable part of the Cava which hath a power of contraction, somewhat like a muscular power. In frogs, and animals that have cold blood, that part of the Cava which goeth out of the liver, hath (*b*) a pulsation, as also its branches, from this going off, even to the heart, the Superior Cava, which extends beyond the lungs to the head and neighbouring parts, and even to both the brachial veins, have a motion of contraction very sensible, by the assistance of which they convey the blood into the auricle; the contraction of the Vena Cava takes place also

(*a*) These experiments are to be found in their order in the 17th section of the second dissertation on Irritability.

(*b*) It giveth two branches to this viscus, and the third descends the length of the lower belly

some-

sometimes under the liver, especially if the Aorta is tied, according to nature the motion of the Vena Cava always preceeds the contraction of the auricle. In a dog, and in animals like man, the Vena Cava, and especially its superior trunk, hath a power of contraction, as there is also, though less sensible, in the Inferior Cava, even to the Diaphragm and liver, for I speak not here on that motion, which depends on respiration. I have observed in a dog, this motion of the Vena Cava to remain full five hours after death. It is therefore certain that the motion of the heart begins by the contraction of the Vena Cava, which drives the blood into the right auricle by true pulsations. Old experiments made me suspect this, and I am convinced thereof by repeating them. As the right ear is larger than both the Cavæ, it makes no resistance to the blood, which it receives from them, it swells by degrees, and, when its distension is increased to a certain degree, the irritation which it occasions, pronuceth a motion in the auricle. I have often seen the motion of the auricle to begin at the blind sack which lieth on the Aorta, and descend towards the inferior part. I have also observed the part which is on the right side in man, to draw near that part which is on the left, and reciprocally the left also to be brought towards the

the right; and the convexity, which is between the right and left extremities of the auricle, to lower itself at every pulsation. Its constriction is composed of all these before-mentioned motions.

In a dead subject, by pressing the auricle, we make the blood re-pass partly into the ventricle, and partly into one of the Cavæ, there being no valves between these veins and the right auricle, and the valves which are at the entrance of the jugular vein being apparently too weak to resist the effort of the blood.

Without doubt, in the common order of the circulation, both the Cavæ resist the blood of the auricle by the pressure of that which they themselves contain, by reason of which resistance it is discharged into the right ventricle. For the jugular vein doth not appear to have any pulsation in a man in health, or in any animal at rest: but when a man exerts his strength, or whose blood by any cause whatever passeth with difficulty into the lungs, it appears by the swelling of the neck or face, that some blood re-passeth from the auricle into the jugulars, and apparently into the Venæ Cavæ; perhaps this is generally the reason of the largeness of the neck, which many women have after delivery, and which is too frequent in my country. An ancient presage of the Romans seems founded upon

upon this obfervation. 'Tis true that they extended too far their opinion concerning this enlarged fize of the neck. I have very diftinctly obferved the blood to re-pafs into the Mammaries, the fubclavians, and other veins: and this I am now obferving in a cat, which is an animal very vigorous.

'Tis known that, in a dying animal, the auricle contracts itfelf, and palpitates more frequently than the ventricle, and that it hath fometimes three, four, and even fix contractions during one fyftole of the heart. Perhaps, at this time, the auricle cannot propel blood enough into the heart, fo as to excite a motion by way of a ftimulus, after many contractions; and, perhaps, the blood, thickened in thefe laft moments, paffeth no more to the ventricle, which often happens in dogs which have a very vifcid blood. I have feen the right auricle fo filled with this blood, that thereby it loft intirely its irritability and power of contraction, which happens to the bladder when too full of urine, and the fame phænomenon appeared, whether this coagulation was naturally formed, or whether I had occafioned it by any acid injection. I have alfo feen the fuperior appendix, with much labour, endeavouring to defcend, without being able to difcharge its blood; at which time the inferior part of the auricle was at reft.

Moreover, the contractile power of this auricle preserves itself generally very long; because, after the cessation of motion in the left ventricle, cold, weight, and other causes, continue to determine the blood towards this auricle, wherein much is generally found after death, and it is the common seat of Polypus's.

I have observed its last motion to be made in the inferior part, at the insertion of the Abdominal Cava, at other times, the appendix is the last in motion. The right ventricle being filled with blood, extends itself, recovers, enlargeth itself, and, stimulated by the blood, even contracts itself, in the following manner: its motion descends from the base towards the division of the ventricles, at the same time the parieties approach each other, and the cavity diminisheth. On opening the ventricle at this time, I have clearly observed, that the tendons of the valves were relaxed; the same appeared on opening the left ventricle. At this time the heart resists the finger, when it is brought into contact with it outwardly, and binds it when it is introduced into its cavity. In a cat, these motions are performed with but little force.

When the animal begins to languish, the right ventricle seldom contracts itself, and in an imperfect manner, and its motions degenerate into particular tremors of small portions of of flesh, which have distinct motions of palpitation in the middle of other portions of flesh which are at rest, the last motion is made at the Apex.

From the right ventricle, all the blood naturally passeth into the pulmonary artery, with more force than is generally supposed; for I have seen, in a dog, the blood of this artery to spring to the same height as that of the Aorta. In a dying animal, the valves of the veins do not exactly meet and close; and a great part of the blood of the right ventricle re-passeth into its auricle. I have observed also in a living cat, that the blood returned into the auricle by pressing the heart. In frogs, we observe very distinctly for some hours, the blood and air to pass from the auricle into the ventricle, and from the ventricle into the auricle, which is a proof that the valves do not exactly close: it is also as certain, that in a living animal, all that part of the blood of the ventricle contained between the venal valve and the auricle, doth not re-enter the auricle at every contraction of the heart, as Rouhault hath justly observed (c).

The motion of this ventricle subsists much longer than that of the left, but not so long as the right ear, which is almost always the last part in which the blood collects.

(c) Offervationi fisiche Anatomiche, p. 80

We shall not trace the blood of the pulmonary artery in its course through the lungs; it is sufficient to say, that, at its return, it is received into the left sinus, and into the small appendix of this sinus, called the auricle. This auricle, in contracting itself, descends towards its base, and becomes shorter in emptying itself: I only once observed the auricle and the left sinus only to straiten themselves without becoming shorter; so that the posterior pariety touched the anterior, and the point of the auricle did not descend.

This auricle hath something particular, which is, that it trembles and palpitates with a much greater swiftness than the right auricle, although the intire contractions are not more frequent than those of the latter.

The motion of this auricle ceaseth, and it loseth its irritability before the ventricles, if the blood is not intirely coagulated in the parts of the heart on the right side, or if the Aorta is not tied up: for, having coagulated the blood by an injection with vinegar, not only the left auricle continued its motions, even after the right, but moreover it became at that time the only part in which we could recal the suppressed motions. I read before you, gentlemen, since the year 1751, expements with respect to a ligature on the Aorta, and

and its effects on the left auricle (*d*). It is not to be doubted, that in a living animal in health, the left auricle dischargeth itself into the ventricle of the same side, but doth any part of its blood pass again into the pulmonary vein? This I will not decide: analogy seems to persuade it, from what is observed with respect to the right auricle and Vena Cava in animals that are near death; but the situation of the sinus makes it very difficult to observe it exactly.

The left ventricle deserves more particularly to be called the heart, since the septum and the greatest part of the Apex of the heart properly belongs to it, and makes only one body with it; also it moves different from the right ventricle: for, its fleshy fibres re-ascend all intire from the point, the origine of motion being there, from whence it proceeds towards the superior part and towards the septum, and the whole heart, as I have observed in a cat, ascends towards its base and towards the Aorta: at which time the fleshy parieties approach each other, and straiten the cavity of this ventricle. During this motion, all the fleshy fibres of the heart become wrinkled by transverse folds, the same is observed in the right ventricle. At this time the pulmonary artery and Aorta are

(*d*) Comment. tom 1 p 273, and the following, it is the small dissertation re-printed after this.

drawn downwards. The strength of this ventricle a little exceeds that of the right.

The principle, and almost sole cause, why the point of the heart is thrust forward, is the situation of the left sinus. When we inflate this sinus, after having opened the breast, the point of the heart is seen briskly to draw near the nipple. In frogs, the auricle is placed behind the heart, and it is found in its diastole, when the heart is in its systole. Its motion also contributes to move the point of the heart forwards: but whether the Aorta be full or empty, it doth not appear that this produceth any change in the situation of the heart in this animal.

The point of the heart preserves its irritability very long, and keeps in motion longer than all the other parts of this ventricle. I have observed the septum to tremble and palpitate, after all the parts of the heart, and even the auricles, were intirely at rest. Moreover, I have observed sometimes in cats, the cessation of motion to begin at the left auricle, and afterwards it took place in the ventricle on the same side, and also after this in the right ventricle, at a time when the right ear appeared the last in motion.

This is the place to examine whether the point of the heart recedes from, or approacheth its base in the systole. I will not quote all the authors that have treated on this

this matter It is sufficient for me to be able to assert, that in a very great number of experiments made on dogs, cats, kids, sheep, rabbits, mice, hedge hogs (e), hogs, and frogs, I have constantly seen, that at the time of the contraction of the left ventricle, the point of the heart raiseth itself, and, approaching the base, comes into contact with the breast; but, in the diastole, as the ventricle fills, the heart lengthens itself, and extends itself in a very sensible manner. I have seen in a frog, which is a very little animal, this point to draw near the sternum a whole line in the systole, and the heart consequently to bend in proportion. and, in the same animal, I have observed this contraction and shortening, at a time when the systole sensibly appeared, although the arteries were tied up, and, consequently, no blood could go out from the heart.

The eel, whose heart is particularly formed, is larger below, and terminates in a point near the Aorta, is the only animal, whose heart can be said to lengthen itself at the time of its contraction, for it extends its point from the Aorta below as far as the liver. at the time it conveys its blood

---

(e) Permit me here to say, as I have an occasion to speak of this animal, that in it I always found a Pericardium and its blood warm, although the contrary hath been asserted.

into the Aorta. M. Queye (*f*) hath obferved this in the tortoife, and I cannot fay whether the ftructure of its heart is the fame with that of the eel

This motion of conftriction compreffeth the blood of the left ventricle, into which, on introducing the finger, a compreffion may be perceived, as I have before related with refpect to the right ventricle

If the point of the heart is cut at this time, the blood is driven from the ventricle. This blood is naturally propelled into the Aorta, which becomes fwelled, and, efpecially, if the artery was before tied up: for the heart, irritated by this ligature, labours ftrongly to free itfelf from its contained blood, and the number and force of the pulfations increafe even in the eel, which is a cold and fluggifh animal (*g*)

When the heart is abfolutely empty, it remains intirely at reft, and, its folds difappearing, its furface becomes fmooth; and, in this ftate, which is called relaxation in the mufcles, it becomes foft, extended, ftrait, and at reft. It remains in this indolent ftate without recovering its fyftole, not only for minutes, but when the animal is in a languifhing ftate for whole half hours. This continuance of a ftate of reft is alone suffi-

(*f*) Differt de Syncope
(*g*) See the differtation of M Remus, p 22.

cient to prove, that the diastole is not an effect of muscular action, but of relaxation and weakness. A muscular contraction hath never continued whole half hours.

A ligature on the Aorta doth not prevent, in the heart of a frog, the same symptoms which it hath in a state of rest, the heart extends, unites, and lengthens itself: it recovers again its state of diastole, although it remains full of blood.

Moreover, the heart doth not become red at the time of the diastole, neither doth it become pale at the time of the systole; and repeated experiments have convinced me, that all which Harvey hath wrote, with respect to its changing its colour, only takes place in animals that have cold blood, in which we are able to trace by the eye, a column of blood, which appears successively in the Vena Cava, in the auricle, in the heart, and in the Aorta, all which parts become red the time this red column is passing them, and become white when it passed off; but neither the flesh of the heart, nor of the muscles, suffer any change in their colour, whether the heart is in a state of rest, or in a state of contraction.

The blood propelled into the Aorta is from thence distributed into all parts of the animal, but if the Aorta is tied up, I have seen it return into the heart, which proves, that in a living animal, the effect of the valves is not of so great a consequence as is supposed.

Therefore the Vena Cava, the two auricles, and afterwards the two ventricles, are successively contracted in the order above-related, and become relaxed in the same order, so that the dilatation, or the contraction of the Vena Cava, and of the two ventricles, always happen at the same instant of time. 'Tis an agreeable sight to observe the gradation which ensues on the filling of these parts, in an animal that hath cold blood: at first, part of the auricle on the right side, which is behind the heart, swells with blood, afterwards the part on the left side of this auricle; afterwards the ventricle, and, lastly, the artery, which goes off from the heart, passing obliquely before the auricle: this I have observed for nine hours.

Experiment falsified all that hath been wrote with respect to the alternate contraction of the two auricles or ventricles. The authors of this hypothesis have made the right ventricle to contract itself before the left, and the celebrated Dr. Nicols (*h*), and Lancisi (*i*), have been both deceived: the former hath made this difference of one pulsation, and the other only of part of a pulsation.

(*h*) Compend Oeconom p 27
(*i*) De Corde & Aneurismat prepos 59, 60, 61.

But,

But, on opening both the ventricles, the blood makes intirely, at the same time, two currents from the two ventricles. It is sufficiently known, that the heart is very irritable; but nothing better discovers this truth, or revives its motions with such certainty as the air; and its motion continue much longer, when they are produced by inflating the heart, than when they depend on the blood which it contains: also, in a dying animal, it recovereth again, by its own power, its motions, after it had been in a perfect state of rest; and, after some contractions of the right auricle, it seems to recover in such a manner, that the intervals between these different revived motions, become always longer. The whole heart, in a living animal, hath one common motion; and when the ribs ascend in inspiration, the heart sinks with the Diaphragm, and ascends again at the time of expiration. Also the Venæ Cavæ are drawn by the Diaphragm, and descend at the time of inspiration. Those who believe that part of the Diaphragm which supports the heart immoveable, seem never to have opened living animals. The contractile force of the arteries is generally considered as the second cause of the motion of the blood. Many authors suppose this power equal to that of the heart; and others believe it more con-

considerable (*k*). Many believe that the force of the heart is sufficient to propel the blood, even into the small arteries; and that the force of the arteries is the cause of its return into the veins (*l*). On this reasoning, a want of pulse in the veins is commonly accounted for. It is believed that the venal blood, being alternatively propelled by the force of the heart, and by that of the arteries, preserves an uniform motion without intermission (*m*). We find in animals that have warm blood, and in man, that the arteries, even the smallest branches of the brain, have red fibres, susceptible of contraction, and capable of causing a constriction, and this force is proved by experiments. When an artery is tied up, the part under the ligature propels equally into the veins it contained blood (*n*). If two ligatures are made on the artery, the blood contained between the two passeth equally into the neighbouring branches (*o*) When the Aorta is ossified, the Vena Cava becomes filled with blood coagulated and im-

---

(*k*) M Senac This celebrated physician believed, that not only the force of the arteries preserve the force of the heart which dilates them, but also that it multiplieth it. Traite du Cœur, tom ii p. 166 See p. 199, 200 224, 225, &c.
(*l*) Pechlin de Corde, N° 21 Thomson Dissertat. i Morisson on the Choice of Bleeding
(*m*) M Sauvage Pulsus Theor p 26
(*n*) Drelincourt Canicid 1 Pecquet p 46.
(*o*) Schwenke Hæmatolog p 80

moveable

moveable (*p*). We have other experiments of this kind.

Although I have no thoughts of refuting these facts, I think it becomes me to report what anatomy and experiments have taught me with respect to this matter. In the first place, the arteries of frogs have always appeared to me destitute of any power of contraction, when I considered the perfect equality of their diameter in the state of inanition and repletion, or when I examined the effects which poisons made on them, the most corroding of which have never been able to produce in them the least contraction (*q*); and, on observing their composition, which is much like the cellular net-work, and which hath not any one fleshy fibre; and, lastly, on reflecting on their want of pulse, since it appears that the vessels which have no dilatation, have consequently no contraction, and that the arteries and veins of frogs, touched with spirit of nitre, have suffered no change, neither do they contract themselves: although this poison produceth even a change of the blood in the vessels, and gives it an earthy colour, and of the consistence of dirt, nothing in a manner can be concluded from the inanition of the vessels. In frogs, the arte-

(*p*) Sanctorini de Nutritione
(*q*) See in the Dissertation of M. Remus, p. 48. The experiments which we made together.

ries are often intirely empty, and after bleedings, under the ligatures, and in other circumstances, we observe the globules of blood gradually to forsake the artery, until it becomes intirely empty and white. These vessels empty themselves so intirely, that not one single globule remains, but I have been convinced, by many experiments, that the globules are moved in the arteries in these cases, even without any contraction of the vessels, and independent of the force of the heart. In an artery almost empty, one single row of globules is observed, at the extremity of the artery, to advance, to stop, to move in a contrary direction, and at last to disappear, so that the best microscopes are not able to discover the smallest motion in the vessels, or any diminution in the diameter of the artery, after the blood hath left it.

With respect to the arteries of animals that have warm blood, and which have an apparent pulse, I agree that they have strength sufficient to recover themselves after they have been dilated, this strength depends on the circular muscular fibres.

But we shall be easily convinced, even in this species of animals, that the force of the heart is very superior to that of the arteries, if we consider what follows. First, with respect to the early force of the heart in the first times of a fœtus. This organ propels
the

the blood through gelatinous arteries. We may live very long, although almost all the arteries are ossified, since we find often in dead subjects, a continuation of bony Laminæ from the head to the foot, between the muscular and internal coat of the arteries of people, who, when living, followed their business, and complained of no indisposition depending on the irregularity of the circulation (r). For, although in the end a sphacelus terminates this state, when the arteries are no longer susceptible of any dilatation, yet they may live many years before a sphacelus ensues; and these old men, whose arteries have thus become ossified, used the exercise of walking at this time, have had a pulse, preserved their natural warmth, and followed their business a considerable time. Nobody will suppose, that a degeneration like this, can be the work of a small time, and it is manifest that much time is required to give a glutinous liquor the hardness of a bone. We must yet compare the great irritability of the heart, which inflation, or every other

(r) This is frequent enough in old men. Harvey relates two examples, de Circulat. Sanguinis, p. 218, without mentioning any inconvenience in the life-times of these men. The case which I have observed, may be seen in the Philosophical Transactions, N° 483. Opuscul Patholog Observat. 46. 52. and those which other authors have observed in the Philosophical Transactions, N° 299.

mechanical irritation, procures, with the perfect Inertia and weakness of the arteries, which may be irritated in a living animal by the knife, the needle, poison, or by any other means, without their contracting themselves the least in the world (s). Lastly, it must be considered, that the motion of the blood recovers itself again in a man that hath been drowned, and this only by irritating the heart. If the heart alone is able to make the blood circulate, in immoveable vessels, in animals that have cold blood; in animals that have warm blood, which have proportionably a heart much larger than the others (t), it will be able more easily to produce a circulation without any foreign help.

I speak not here of the mechanical contraction of arteries that are dried up, or of the effect resulting therefrom. as the membranes become dry, they either express and discharge their blood, or they change it into

(s) Comment. Societ. Reg. Gott. tom. II. p. 131. 141. Dissertation on the irritable and sensible Parts, sect. 11.

(t) Robinson, of Food and Discharges, saith, that in using the mean terms, the heart of a cow, of a bird, and of a fish, is in the following proportion, $\frac{1}{283}$, $\frac{1}{175}$, $\frac{1}{136}$. That is to say, that proportions considered relative to the mass of the animal, the heart of a very slow quadruped is more than five times larger than that of fish. Confront p. 107 with p. 120.

fibres

fibres and membranes, and the artery becomes filled with a cellular marrow, but these changes take their rise from dead force, and continue their action for years after the circular fibres have lost theirs: an example whereof we have in the umbilical arteries, in the arterial canal, and in Aneurisms.

Of this nature, I suppose that force which makes an artery that is cut, to shrink *(u)*; and which is yet stronger and more sensible in the tendons or ligaments, although they are neither hollow nor irritable.

Also the motion of the muscles is reckoned one of the powers that help the circulation, which acts chiefly on the veins; but I speak not here of that motion, by which it is said, even by the most modern authors, that the blood is driven from the muscle during its contraction. For, having often examined with a microscope, the intestines and the great muscle on the leg of a frog, at the time of their contraction, I have observed that, in in these parts, the blood is seen in them, and moves in their vessels, both before the contraction and in the following relaxation, and that the arteries remain equally full, both at the one time and the other; but the time of the contraction is so short, and the focus of the microscope so suddenly changeth, that I

(u) M. de Sauvage Theor. Tumor p. 8.

know

know not any method to obferve a mufcular fibre at the inftant of its contraction. Alfo, the argument that is made ufe of to ground this hypothefis is (*x*) taken from a ftrong current of blood, on moving the arm at the time of bleeding; but this does not prove what they would infer from it For, whoever hath obferved the rapidity with which they force the blood out of the vein, by compreffing and turning in their hand any cylindrical inftrument, cannot be perfuaded that this blood was expreffed at this moment of time, from the capillary arteries of thefe mufcles into the veins and venal trunks, and, laftly, into the vein that is opened by the furgeon Moreover, an experiment very eafy, and which may be repeated on any animal, proves that the mufcles do not become pale when they act, which muft happen if their blood left them at this time. All this fyftem is founded (*y*) on Harvey before cited; and, through an inconfiderate analogy, they have attributed to all the mufcles a property which is peculiar to the heart, as it is a refervoir of blood, but not as it is a mufcle.

But the mufcles contribute, in a different manner, to the circulation of the blood: they comprefs the veins which lie between them,

(*x*) Memoire fur le Mouvement des Mufcles, N° 20 p 82 Recueil pour le Prix de l'Academie
(*y*) Pages 22 and 23

and

and this compression, whose effect is directed by the valves, contributes to hasten the blood from the seat of the heart. This is the true cause why the force of the blood, at the time of bleeding, is increased, by moving in the hand some instrument, or by muscular efforts of the wrist; it is also the cause of a phænomenon often mentioned by Boerhaave: that is to say, when the lower belly of an animal is opened, the vessels of the Mesentery and of the intestines fill with blood, so as to become almost varicous, by having lost this auxiliary contraction which the muscles of the lower belly produced in them. It is this effect of muscular motion, which is the cause that nobody can deprive himself of it for any considerable time, without suffering a diminution of the circulation, especially in the feet, and which would produce in them a continual coldness and an œdema: from hence I account for the stones, which are so frequently found in the gall-bladder of criminals which have been a long time in gaol, and many other the like phænomena.

I have with care examined a particular muscle, to satisfy myself in what manner it assists the circulation of the blood, I mean the Diaphragm. The late M. Walther having opposed what I had advanced concerning the force this muscle useth in binding the Vena Cava, I made a great number of experiments

riments on dogs, cats, and other like animals; and I obferved, after having opened the lower belly, that, at the time of infpiration, the ribs afcend, and the Diaphragm defcends; and that, by this motion, the Vena Cava is drawn down and conftringed, fo as to empty itfelf and become pale. and it is evident that the fame thing muft more reafonably take place, if the lower belly is not opened, and that its cavity being intire full, all the parts are brought more into contact. The moment following, when the Diaphragm becomes relaxed, the Vena Cava re-afcends, and becomes filled with blood, which returns from the Abdomen This motion is fo apparent, that I fhould have attributed to it the phæromena which I have obferved in the brain, and which I have fet forth elfewhere, if I had not obferved the fame changes to have happened in the arm and neck, which are parts to which this action of the Diaphragm cannot extend. This remark difcovers to us a new effect of refifting powers, which is that, by reafon of the length of infpiration, they hinder the return of the blood from the inferior parts of the lower belly.

I have formerly treated on the effect the nerves have on the arteries. M. Mekel hath lately treated on the fame (z) M. Senac be-

(z) Memoires de l'Acad Roy de Berlin, 1751 The tide is 1752

lieves

lieves this effect very confiderable; and that the nerves have a power of extending and relaxing the arteries (*a*), to ftop the motion of the blood in the very fmall ones (*b*), and to produce other the like phænomena.

It is certain, that confiderable nerves are found near the carotid and its large branches, but we cannot prove that they make a part of, or are diftributed into, the fubftance of the arteries, fince the arteries in general are almoft infenfible, and may be tied up in man and animals without pain. On the other hand, the fudden changes produced in the circulation by the mind, the erection of the Penis, of the Clitoris, of the nipples of the breaft; the changes of colour in the cheeks; Cold and heat, Tremors, Inflammations, Obftructions, the ftrong motions which violent pains or wounds of the nerves often occafion. All thefe facts confidered, render very probable the action of the nerves on the arteries; fince it by this appears, that they have certainly a great power, either of retarding or accelerating the circulation.

But I have never been able by any experiment, to find by obfervation, that irritating the nerves created any change in the velocity of the humours contained in the veffels of the

---

(*a*) Traité du Cœur, tom. ii. p 108. 209.
(*b*) Ibid. p 170.

circulation. I have indeed obferved, once or twice, that, by irritating the nerves, it revived the action of the blood, and reftored the motion of it in arteries that were cut, which had ceafed to fupply any. But I have had great reafon to attribute this effect to fome mechanical action (c) By irritating the phrenic nerve in large animals, I have never found that the pulfations of the heart became altered, and another obfervation, which is very material, is, that in hyfteric paroxyfms, in the Tetanos and Emproftotonos, often the pulfe is neither increafed or altered, notwithftanding the violent agitations the nerves and mufcles undergo. Moreover, by irritating the fpinal marrow, all the mufcles become convulfed, the heart excepted, which preferves its regular motions, if the fpinal marrow is deftroyed, the heart preferves its motion, and it continues to move in a frog after the head is cut off (d), but enough of this here.

Heat and co'd are almoft the only agents on the nutritious juice of vegetables, heat makes it afcend, and cold the contrary It is eafily obferved in men, that the cold air makes their hands pale, dry, and rough, that it forceth back all the blood, not only from the fmall cutaneous veffels, but alfo from the large

(c) Malpighi relates that a convulfion had reftored the courfe of the blood Oper Pofthum p 92
(d) Redi hath obferved it in a tortoife.

veins on the back of the hand; and at length when all the blood is withdrawn, the whole part perisheth, and remains only a white insensible mass (e). It is to the cold air, which binds and shortens every thing in nature, that I attribute the collections of blood that are sometimes observed in the Vena Cava and right ventricle: for, since it is proved by the experiments of the celebrated M. Clifton Wintringham, that, in the animal body, the branches are every-where more dense and firm, proportionally as their trunks, the same cause acting on all the vessels, the effect of these constrictions will be greater in the small vessels, which are the more firm, and less in the large trunks which are more lax, and the force of the small vessels prevailing, they will empty themselves into the great trunks I do not speak here concerning this effect of cold on the vessels of respiration nor on the skin, which it hardens, so as to make it change the direction of its hairs; my thoughts whereof I shall reserve for my physiology.

Heat, on the contrary, relaxeth and resolves every thing: it seemeth to dilate the vessels, and make them more easily give way to the action of the blood, and increase their diameter, which may be observed in the cutaneous veins of the hands. A greater quantity of blood is drove into the heated parts,

(e) Ellis's Voyage to Hudson's Bay, p. 176

which make the less resistance, for the member swells and becomes red, either on being suspended in warm water, or heated by frictions. On warming the vessels of a frog, in which there is any coagulated blood, the coagulum dissipates, and the disengaged globules go off from the parieties, an experiment which Lewenhoeck hath accurately made on a bat, and which I have verified (*f*), but I have not made any fresh experiments with respect to these causes of the variation of motions. I shall now more fully speak as to the effects of weight. It is not surprising, that this force contributes to determine the motion of the blood, not only after death, but even during life, as the blood is heavier than water, whose gravity alone produceth so great a motion in mechanical tubes. Andrew Pasta (*g*), an eminent physician at Bergama, hath very exactly observed, and also very well described, the effects produced after death by the weight of the blood. I have examined the effects of this force on living frogs. My motive for this examination was partly because eminent men, and whom I respect, have denied that this weight had any influence on the circulation in living animals (*h*). This experiment is very

(*f*) Experim. & Contemp. tom. ii. p. 108.
(*g*) De Motu Sanguinis post Mortem.
(*h*) A. F. Walther de Acceleratione & Retardatione Sanguinis.

easily

eafily made. we need only elevate and lift up the whole Mefentery, having taken care not to wound it, and all the veins will be found to empty themfelves, and to look like white threads; loofe it, and leave the fame veffels to their own weight, and the body of the frog becoming higher than the Mefentery, you will find all the veins to fill themfelves with blood, and to receive again their red colour. ufe a microfcope, and obferve fome current that is perpendicular to the board on which the animal is extended, turn afterwards the whole machine upfide down, that its inferior extremity become the fuperior. obferve again, and you will apparently find this torrent of blood inverted, and to move in a contrary direction to what you had obferved, and to defcend inftead of afcending. This is eafily repeated, it becomes more apparent after the animal is dead, or when in a languifhing ftate: but the circulation in the veins is never ftrong enough, fo as not to undergo an alteration by the refiftance of the weight. This effect of gravitation appears but little in the arterial blood, unlefs its motion hath began to abate; in that cafe it becomes retrograde, and is propelled by its weight. By this we fee that, even in a living animal in health, the venal blood very eafily moves, as its weight directs it, and with a greater difficulty in the contrary direction;

rection, and that sometimes, in this case, it falls again towards the parts it comes from. This teacheth us the true cause of the Incubus, and of that heavy drowsiness of a person that sleepeth lying on his back, or that sleepeth in a perfect level; for his blood ascends to the head more easily than it would in a situation not so strait, and it returns from thence with more difficulty, because it is not assisted in its return by the force of its weight Thus we see why the feet are subject to Varices, to œdematous tumours; and why they become cold the fi st, although covered These effects are p oduced, because the blood returns with difficulty from the inferior parts of the body, from whence it must ascend, contrary to the force of its gravity

From hence also we may easily comprehend why the soothsayers among the Romans, observing the flight of birds had varicous legs Why printers, and other tradesmen, are subject to œdematous legs. Why the blood flies to the eyes of people that read small characters, or who employ themselves in work that is extremely fine. This defluxion of humours on the eyes extends them, making the Cornea protuberant, and these people become what we term Myopes. We see also why those who stoop much in reading, are subject to a troublesome rheume of the head, created by a stoppage of the blood in the vessels of the nose. We discover also by this same phænomenon, the necessity of the valves in the limbs, especially in the feet, whereby the blood of the Abdomen is hindered from resisting, by its gravity and weight, the return of the blood from the feet, either in sitting, walking, or standing. I have before taken notice, that I have not been able to discover any valve in frogs, nor in the human Mesentery, which is the cause of the hæmorhoides. I do not believe any author hitherto hath proved by facts, the power that gravity and weight hath of retarding in a living animal the motion of the blood, or of giving it a retrograde motion.

The air dilating itself in the blood after death, occasions various motions (1). I have often, after having broke the bronchial vessels, observed it to disperse itself through the Trachea and mouth, especially in women dying in childbed, or in others dying of some sudden and malignant fever: this probably is the only cause of the Vampyrs. It is certain, that I have seen the blood that was found in the heart of a young man filled with air, to resolve itself into froth, and to discharge itself from the opening I had made in the heart. At another time I saw the blood to discharge itself from the mouth of a very fine woman, who died in

(1) Lancisci de subitanea morte, I. C. p. 16.

child-

childbed, so as to fill the shroud. Thus Schurig hath observed in an apoplectical person, the blood to come out of the mouth with much froth and noise (*k*) Hildanus hath also seen blood discharge itself from the mouth of one that had been drowned, sixteen hours after his death (*l*). Cases of this nature may be found every-where and, perhaps, this is the only cause of the bleeding in dead people, which the superstition of the ancients hath regarded as an index of divine vengeance, which discovered the criminal by this bleeding his presence had created in the body of the person he had deprived of life It is to this expansion of the air, produced by putrefaction, that deliveries which have happened to women after their deaths, are to be attributed.

The last article that remains for me to treat of, and which deserves being more amply considered, is the motion of the blood, which continues after the heart is taken away, or the Aorta tied up, and which does not belong to any of the preceding causes. I have made for this purpose thirty-three experiments: in fifteen I have cut off the heart, and, in seventeen, the two great branches of the Aorta; and in these last experiments I performed this operation without being able to observe any change in the veins But,

(*k*) Sialographia, p. 405. (*l*) Cent 3 Obs 12

before me, Woodward had obferved the motion of the blood to continue for ten minutes in the tail of a little fifh that had been cut off (*m*).

Borelli was the firft who taught us, that, after the heart was deftroyed, the blood gradually removed out of the arteries, until they became abfolutely empty (*n*), after having taken away the heart, or, which is the fame with refpect to the arteries, after having cut off the two great branches which the Aorta of frogs fends out at its rife. In twenty-three experiments, the motion ceafed feven times in the arteries of the Mefentery. in eight other cafes, the blood had a retrograde motion, and this retrograde motion was twice very rapid, and continued to a perfect inanition, in four other frogs, the blood balanced for near an hour, going and coming continually from the trunk to the branch, and from the branch to the trunk. Laftly, in the four laft animals, I obferved the fame direction of motion as in the natural ftate, and this natural motion preferved itfelf in a toad for twenty minutes.

We may infer from hence, that, after the heart is taken away, or the great arteries, the arterial blood hath yet continued its motions for a certain time, from fixteen to twenty-one,

(*m*) Supplement p. 102.
(*n*) De Motu Animalium, lib. 2. prop. 31.

twenty-seven, thirty, and thirty-six minutes, the more frequently it hath had an oscillatory motion, less frequently a retrograde one, and only once it continued to move in its natural order.

Bleeding five times restored the motion of the blood as in a living animal, so that when there was but very few globules in the artery, if, at that time, this operation was performed even fifteen minutes after the heart was cut off, the artery filled itself again with blood, which came at first very readily, and even against the force of its weight, but afterwards more slowly

I have examined the motion of the venal blood in twenty-two animals, after having cut off the heart: in thirteen, it preserved itself in its natural direction, for twelve to seventeen minutes, in three others it took a retrograde motion, and returned from the Mesentery to the intestines, twice it began at first to balance itself. I have observed four times both these motions to take place all at once in different branches, and, in one of these cases, to continue for thirty minutes. I have seen in a vein which had three branches, the small number of globules which remained in one of these branches, to move to and from the intestines in another branch, the blood ascended sufficiently swift towards the heart for fifteen minutes, and afterwards re-

returned in an oscillatory motion; lastly, in the third, it descended also as swiftly from the trunk to the intestine, and returned from thence alternately. I have observed in a toad, that the motion of the blood preserved itself for fifteen minutes after the diminishing of the Aorta; in the capillary network of the veins of the Mesentery, the single globules passed at first into veins of two globules diameter, afterwards into those of three, and from these into the venal trunks.

It hath constantly happened in all these experiments (whereof I have made seventeen) that the blood which had not any motion, recovered itself by bleeding, as in the life-time of the animal, and moved swiftly by the veins of communication, in all directions to the orifice of the vein, and this I observed twenty minutes complete after the death of the animal.

I have seen an oscillation, sufficiently swift in the veins, to arise not only immediately after the death of the animal, but even many minutes after. This motion continued in the veins of communication for twenty-seven, and even for thirty-six minutes; and, in general, whether the heart remained, or was taken away, the branches which join two trunks by an Anastomosis, have always appeared to be the last parts wherein the motion

tion of the blood was preserved, as I have already declared elsewhere

In order to discover the causes of this life without the heart, I first examined if this motion was produced by gravity, I have found also in these experiments, that the oftener the blood moved, not only in the arteries, but also in the veins, against the force of its gravity and weight; that the inversion of the board, on which the animal was extended, did not make any change in the direction of the blood; and that the velocity, with which it is carried towards the vein that is opened, much surpasseth the gravitating power.

It is also very easy to be satisfied, whether this motion depends on the contraction of the vessels I have proved that, in frogs, the vessels have no contraction; I have often seen solitary globules moving in arteries almost empty, and, what is more decisive, I have seen globules that were dispersed between the Laminæ of the Mesentery, to move, oscillate, ascend, and descend, as constantly and as swiftly as those which were included in the vessels. I have seen them ascend and descend along the external parieties of the artery and the sides of the intestines, and, afterwards, after having made a kind of Parabola, to return by a narrower and a more rapid torrent, and distribute themselves between the Laminæ of the Mesentery This motion doth not ab-

abſolutely depend on gravity, and the blood-globules aſcend as ſwiftly as they deſcend; and it is evident that the motion which is performed out of the veſſels does not depend on their contraction.

Doth this motion depend on the ſuction of the ſmall veſſels? Eminent modern phyſicians, ſome of whom are my particular friends (o), have attributed to theſe ſmall veſſels the power of ſuction, by which they draw the blood from the great ones, and they ſuppoſe them capable of aſſiſting the circulation.

But the blood of an animal, whoſe heart is deſtroyed, doth not move only from great veſſels to ſmall ones, but it more frequently moves from the ſmall branches to the great ones. In twelve experiments on the arteries, I have obſerved this laſt motion in eight caſes, and the firſt only in four. The ſame thing takes place with reſpect to the veins: in eighteen experiments, I have obſerved the blood in thirteen animals, to move from the branches to the heart, to balance itſelf in two others, and in only three to turn its courſe from the ſeat of the inteſtines.

I imagine nobody will think it probable that the capillary veins ſhould be able to bring

(o) M. Kenger Phyſiol. German p. 25. This ſentiment is delivered in a diſſertation, whoſe title is, De Suctione Vaſorum Capillarum in Corpore Humano, a Joſ. Brun.

back

back the blood from their trunks, and make it turn its courfe contrary to the natural order of circulation.

For, if nature had given them this power, fhe would have made them inftruments both for the deftruction of the circulation, as of the animal.

What therefore is the caufe of this motion of the blood after death? it is or is not eafy to declare. Let us endeavour to find it. I fee by experiments, that the blood is ftopped by the fides of the Mefentery, and of the membranes, and by the lips of wounds: cut an artery or a vein, 'tis equally the fame, either with the Mefentery, or in the adjacent part of fome confiderable wound of this large membrane, not one drop of blood will come from this opening you have made in the Mefentery. It appears therefore, that the blood is ftrongly attracted by the membranes of the human body. I find alfo that effufed blood conftantly ftops at thefe cellular lines, which every-where accompany the great veffels, and that not only it continues in thefe lines, but that manifeftly it directs itfelf towards them: the fame is true with refpect to the membranes of the inteftines.

I have conftantly obferved that the globules reciprocally attract each other, and that if there was any blood collected in any confiderable arterial trunk, in that cafe, the blood of all the

adjacent

adjacent branches flowed thereto. The same is true with respect to the veins. Also when an Aneurisme is filled with blood, that of the smaller branches moves towards this mass; and if it passeth from thence, it moves on towards some other mass of globules contained in some part of the artery. When the blood is collected in two different places, an oscillation arises between these two kinds of magnetic masses, which attract the globules that are between them, and make them move in opposite directions. The venal branches empty themselves into the trunk, and the blood is a long time balanced and swung by two opposite motions, until at last the force of one prevailing, draws it intirely to itself, or until the vessels become dried up. I once observed, it is true, that the blood which discharged itself from a lacerated vein, and being effused between the Laminæ of the Mesentery, it manifestly had an oscillatory motion, and was absorbed by the vein, and, in a moment after, it was discharged from it again, until this vein and the adjacent branches were filled. The celebrated Dr. Hale hath described the like kind of oscillation in a muscle, whose humours were alternately repelled and attracted by the extremities of the vessels (*p*).

From all these facts, we may, I think, probably conclude, that the blood collects itself

(*p*) Hæmastaticks, p 96.

into

into a mafs in places where there is firft any of this mafs found, and thus it is in all dying animals. For, as to the arteries and veins, all the blood paffeth from the branches into the trunks, and the former empty themfelves, and the latter fill themfelves. therefore the direction of the blood into the veins is the proper and direct motion, and which is the moft frequent; and the motion into the arteries is a retrograde motion, becaufe thefe two different motions tend both equally to bring back the humours into their refpective trunks.

There muft be another caufe for this fwift motion, which carrieth the blood fo conftantly, and with fuch force, towards the openings of wounded veffels, whether it be an invifible and innate contraction of the parieties of the veffels, or fome other property, I know not. Laftly, let what will be the caufes of thefe different motions, it is worth obferving, that forty-one minutes after having cut off the heart, when the blood was intirely in a ftate of reft, I faw frogs make ufe of their mufcles, fo as to jump and make their efcape. This proves that the action of the mufcles doth not depend on the communication of the arteries, nor on any affiftance from the blood. The fame mufcles in the fame frog conftantly tremble by irritating their nerves, and remain always immoveable when they are cut off.

off. This proves that the motion of the muscles continues very strong independent of the arterial blood, but, without the action of the nerves, it is lost. These frogs can see, although their heart is cut off; they draw their eyelids over their eyes, they breathe, and draw the air in at their nostrils, which they can dilate, and give yet other signs of life. The eminent Caldesi hath observed the same in a tortoise, which is an animal analagous enough to frogs (*q*).

Lastly, gentlemen, what is absolutely necessary to be known is, that I made all these experiments, which are very numerous, in the current of these twenty years last, on different kinds of animals. I have sacrificed above eighty that have warm blood, and above seventy that have cold I examined fish with the common microscope of Culpeper, and seldom with the solar one, because I observed that, though it magnifies objects prodigiously, it renders them confused, and their sides not well adjusted. I exposed the frogs on boards, after the manner of Lieberkun (*r*), and I examined them with a glass which did not magnify extremely, yet is preferable to many others for its clearness. I have improved the instru-

(*q*) It lived two days without the heart, p 76. Many of the like examples are found in the Prælect Boerhavian. tom. ii. p 614, 615

(*r*) He hath given a description of them in the Memoirs of the Academy at Berlin of 1745.

ment, by adding a part to keep the glafs as firm as I would have it without the affiftance of the hand.

It is not you, gentlemen, whofe prudence, difcretion, and ability, I acknowledge; but thofe who neither know me, nor the love I have for truth: thefe are the cenfors, I fay, whom I defire not to pafs judgment on my performance, or on the account I give of what I have obferved in one fingle experiment or example. They will find nothing here, neither have they found any thing in my preceding experiments on refpiration, irritability, and fenfiblity, which I have feen once only; I have obferved all with exactnefs, and have verified all more than once. When I faid that the Dura Mater, the tendons, and the Periofteum, had no fenfibility, I knew I oppofed received opinions, which I could not expect would be given up, unlefs nature fhewed herfelf on my fide. When I defcribed the ufes of the internal intercoftals, and proved the abfence of air in the breaft, I knew I fhould find an antagonift in the late M. Hamberger, and that all the medicomathematical fect, which were joined with him with refpect to their opinions, muft take on his fide.

I have only related facts, which, to my fatisfaction, I have proved by repeated experiments,

periments. M. M. Holman, Mecrel, Trendelenbourg, Sidren, Roederer, Sproegel, Oeder, Hahm, Zinn, Ith, Duntz, Runge, De Brunn, have been witnesses, especially of the experiments relative to respiration. I made those proving the absence of air in the breast before the whole society of sciences (s). M. M. Zinn, Walstorf, Dethlef, Remus, Sproegel, Zimmerman, the Baron de Brunn, and many physicians amongst those I have named, have seen those which respect irritability and sensibility (t). M. Remus hath assisted at those which respect the motion of the blood, and any body may see them, if he adds to some patience, a relish for truth, a freedom from prejudice, and a little art. As for those who attack me, after having made one or two experiments, (or perhaps none at all) and unsuccessfully, there are too many criticks, of this stamp, will be convinced of their error, when they attentively examine nature; and they will, with sorrow, find themselves obliged to con-

(s) The fourth of November, 1752. See the Nouvelles Litteraires of Gottingen, of the same month.

(t) M Huerman hath verified at Copenhagen the experiments on the tendons See his Physiolog tom iii. p. 79 and M Tozzetti, Farion, Zinn, Rungf, Pozzi, Andrichi, Muhlman, Emett, and other physicians, have done the same, which will appear in the second volume of Memoirs on the Sensible and Irritable Parts.

fess that they have opposed truth: for, if I want either sufficient health or talents for establishing the truth, I have so good an opinion of mankind, as to assure myself that nature, at some time or other, will find her avengers, who will re-establish her rights on the ruin of prejudice and opinion.

SUPPLEMENT

TO THE

PRECEDING DISSERTATION.

On the Cause of the Motion of the Heart.

Read the tenth day of November, 1751 (*u*).

HOWEVER short this dissertation may be, it will not be without its use. Herein will be seen an experiment, which I have many times made, and which proves that the motion of the heart, and its continual alternate contractions and relaxations, depend on irritation. All the demonstrations that have been hitherto delivered with respect to this phænomenon, are destroyed by human or comparative anatomy.

(*u*) The experiments, on which this dissertation is founded, are contained in the 17th section of the Second Dissertation on the Irritable Parts, and make the experiments 515, and the following to 523.

It is perfectly known, that the right ventricle, especially its auricle, are the last parts of the body preserving motion: experiments taught this to Galen (1), to Harvey (2), and to Boerhaave (3).

I have a long time suspected (4), that the continuance of this motion depended on the blood with which the Venæ Cavæ, contracted by cold and compressed by palpitations and the weight of the muscles, are continually furnishing this ventricle: but the lungs of an animal dying, that are immoveable and collapsed, receive no more blood from the pulmonary artery; and that blood, which its contraction is able to propel into the left auricle, is very little, with respect to that which returns from all the body to the right auricle, to produce any sensible effect. It may then be said, if the right ventricle and its auricle moves longer than the left auricle, that it is because the venal blood supplies them longer.

I resolved to verify my conjecture by experiments, and for this purpose, it was necessary to hinder, if possible, the entrance of the blood into the right ventricle: if by this means its motions ceased, it was a proof that

(1) Admin anatom lib 7 c 15
(2) D ff 1 p 39, 44, &c
(3) Institut re. Med No 159.
(4) Commentar in Boerh t 11 p 609. Pprim Lin. physic, No 113.

they

they depended effectively on the receiving of this blood.

I first tried this experiment by ligatures, because I recollected I had read in Bartholine (5) and in Berger (6), that a ligature on the veins made the motion of the heart cease, and that it recovered itself when the ligature was cut off, and Harvey mentions his having made the same experiment on a serpent (7): but I did not succeed by this method; because, as long as the animal continues warm, the blood that is in the right auricle continues to move it, although none enters it by the Venæ Cavæ; so that after having tied them up in three kittens, the motion of the blood still continued. The same happened to Blanquet, in the experiments related by M. Senac (8). This made me resolve to divide both the cavæ. I had intirely cut them off, but was afraid if I had, that the cessation of the motion of the heart, would be attributed to its want of the continuance of necessary support; after having divided them, I discharged them of all their blood, and tied them up: I afterwards emptied the auricle, whereupon the success of the ex-

(5) Anat. p 376.
(6) De Nat Hum p 62, 63, 306. See also Sorgeloos de Œconom cor. p 66, 69.
(7) L C. p 99
(8) Traité du Cœur. t. 1. p. 449.

periment hath always been certain. When I had taken away all the blood from the auricle, and hindered it from receiving any more, it lost immediately the least appearance of motion, as it is more difficult to empty the ventricle than the auricle, and because it gives way to the impressions which the left ventricle communicates to it; sometimes a small motion may be observed therein, incomparably more feeble than that which it hath when it receives the blood from its auricle and Venæ Cavæ.

I had also an experiment yet more authentic to make. In the natural state, the right ventricle moves longer than the left, because I have said it receives the venal blood longer. In order demonstratively to prove that the blood is effectively the cause of the motion of the heart, I had occasion only to prove, that if the right ventricle and its auricle were deprived of their blood, at a time when the left ventricle was supplied therewith, that the former would thereupon lose their motion, when that of the latter would be preserved

To succeed herein, it seemed at first necessary to empty intirely the right ventricle, by opening the pulmonary artery and the Venæ Cavæ, and to prevent the evacuation of the left ventricle by tying up the Aorta, and afterwards carefully to examine if in this state, the motions of the right ventricle would cease, and

and if thofe of the left ventricle and its auricle were continued.

After fome attempts, which the difficulty of this agreeable undertaking, and the hafty death of the animals had rendered unfuccefsful, the experiment anfwered my defires, the right auricle remained intirely immoveable, and its ventricle preferved only a motion, which was a neceffary confequence of the connexion of its fibres with thofe of the left ventricle, and whereby its exterior parieties were drawn towards the feptum, which divides the two ventricles. The left auricle continued its motion for fome time, the ventricle longer; and I have fometimes obferved, that at the end of two hours it yet contracted itfelf. The experiment thus happily fucceeding, the blood afcended from the point of the left ventricle to the bafe, and afterwards defcended again from the bafe to the point; at which time the right ventricle, if it had any motion, feemed to defcend: at other times I have obferved this in a kid, and it had not any motion at all. This experiment more efpecially fucceeded, when the left auricle emptied itfelf freely into the ventricle, and when the blood had no accefs into the Aorta that was tied up. The point of the left ventricle was always the part which preferved the longeft its motion. Thus may be transferred from the right ventricle to the left, the property of being

being the laſt part of the body in motion, by preſerving a longer time in the latter, the irritation that is produced by the contact of the blood.

A new force is given to this experiment, by endeavouring to inflate the right ventricle by this irritation, it revives and recovers its motions. Moreover, I have always obſerved, that the internal ſurface of the heart, is much more irritable than the external, for, on irritating this by the ſtrongeſt poiſon, the motion communicated to the heart ſoon ended; but, on irritating the internal ſurface only by air, it occaſioned, eſpecially in frogs and even in cats motions that continued very long, although all the parts were become cold I repeated this experiment nine times, in order to preſerve in the left ventricle its motion, when all the other parts had loſt theirs, ſeven times on cats, and twice on kids The reſiſtance and great agitation in dogs, renders them improper for this experiment.

F I N I S.

Lightning Source UK Ltd.
Milton Keynes UK
UKHW032012051222
413454UK00017B/215